FUN WORD LADDERS
GRADE 4-6

SPELLING WORKOUT PUZZLE BOOK
FOR KIDS AGES 9-12

This book includes free bonus that are available here:
www.funspace.club
Follow us: facebook.com/funspaceclub

How to Play

You can start from the bottom or top of the ladder. We give you a first word. Next step will have a hint which not too difficult for children aged 9-12 years. You have to change one letter to be the next word.

For example we play from the top of ladder. The first word is "FISH". The next step we give hint "A hand with the fingers clenched in the palm". Did you guess? It's "FIST". Just change one letter!

See more great books for kids at

www.funspace.club
Follow us : facebook.com/funspaceclub

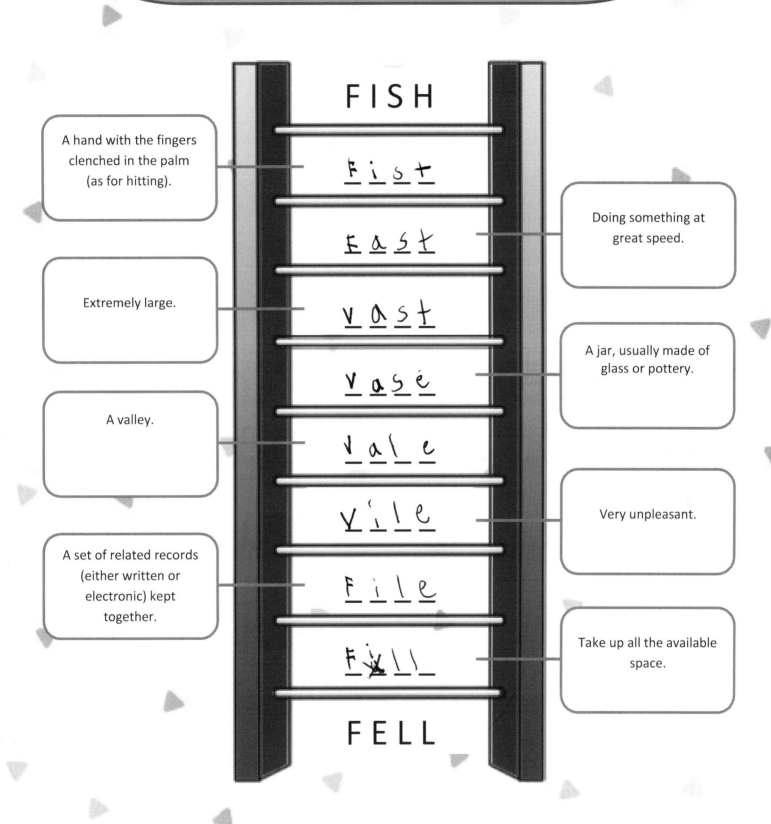

FISH

Fist — A hand with the fingers clenched in the palm (as for hitting).

Fast — Doing something at great speed.

Vast — Extremely large.

Vase — A jar, usually made of glass or pottery.

Vale — A valley.

Vile — Very unpleasant.

File — A set of related records (either written or electronic) kept together.

Fill — Take up all the available space.

FELL

FROM CROSS TO BONES

CROSS

Stupid and does not show consideration for other people.

A yellow-coloured metal made from copper and zinc.

Very troublesome children.

Third-person singular form of the simple present indicative tense of the verb to beat.

Any of various edible seeds of plants of the family Leguminosae used for food. (*Plural form*)

Small pieces of coloured glass, wood, or plastic with a hole through the middle.

Third-person singular form of the simple present indicative tense of the verb to bend.

Third-person singular form of the simple present indicative tense of the verb to bond.

BONES

JUMP

A small, hard swelling that has been caused by an injury or an illness.

_ _ _ _

Walk impeded by some physical limitation or injury.

_ _ _ _

A green fruit that tastes like a lemon.

_ _ _ _

A long thin mark which is drawn or painted on a surface.

_ _ _ _

Lacking companions or companionship.

_ _ _ _

The hard parts inside your body which together form your skeleton.

_ _ _ _

A connection that fastens things together

_ _ _ _

Fearless and daring

_ _ _ _

TOLD

FROM MUNCH TO CLANS

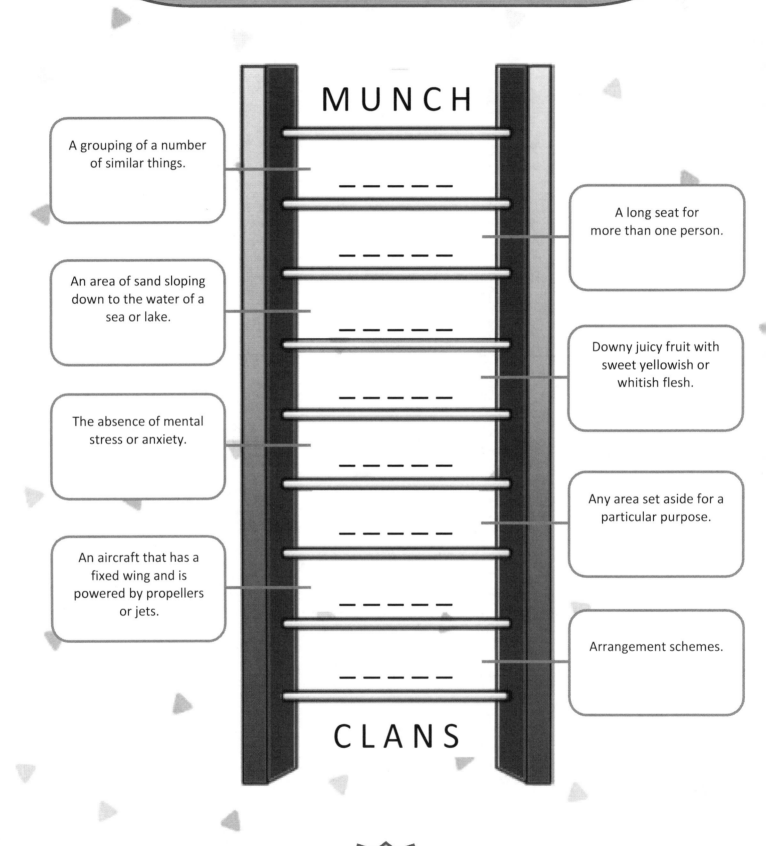

MUNCH

A grouping of a number of similar things.

A long seat for more than one person.

An area of sand sloping down to the water of a sea or lake.

Downy juicy fruit with sweet yellowish or whitish flesh.

The absence of mental stress or anxiety.

Any area set aside for a particular purpose.

An aircraft that has a fixed wing and is powered by propellers or jets.

Arrangement schemes.

CLANS

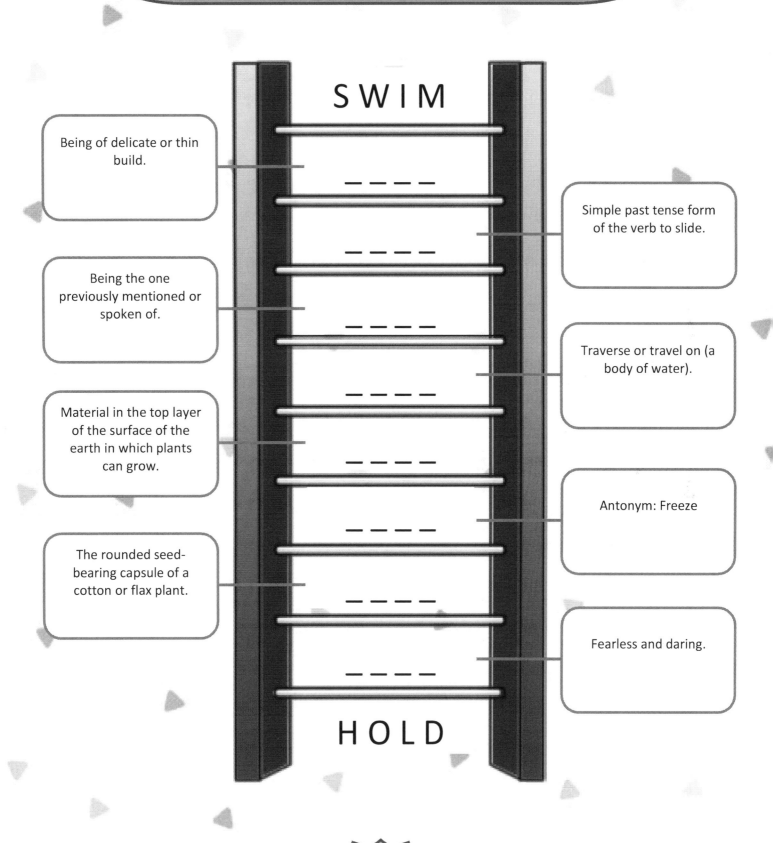

SWIM

Being of delicate or thin build.

Simple past tense form of the verb to slide.

_ _ _ _

Being the one previously mentioned or spoken of.

_ _ _ _

Traverse or travel on (a body of water).

Material in the top layer of the surface of the earth in which plants can grow.

_ _ _ _

Antonym: Freeze

The rounded seed-bearing capsule of a cotton or flax plant.

_ _ _ _

Fearless and daring.

_ _ _ _

HOLD

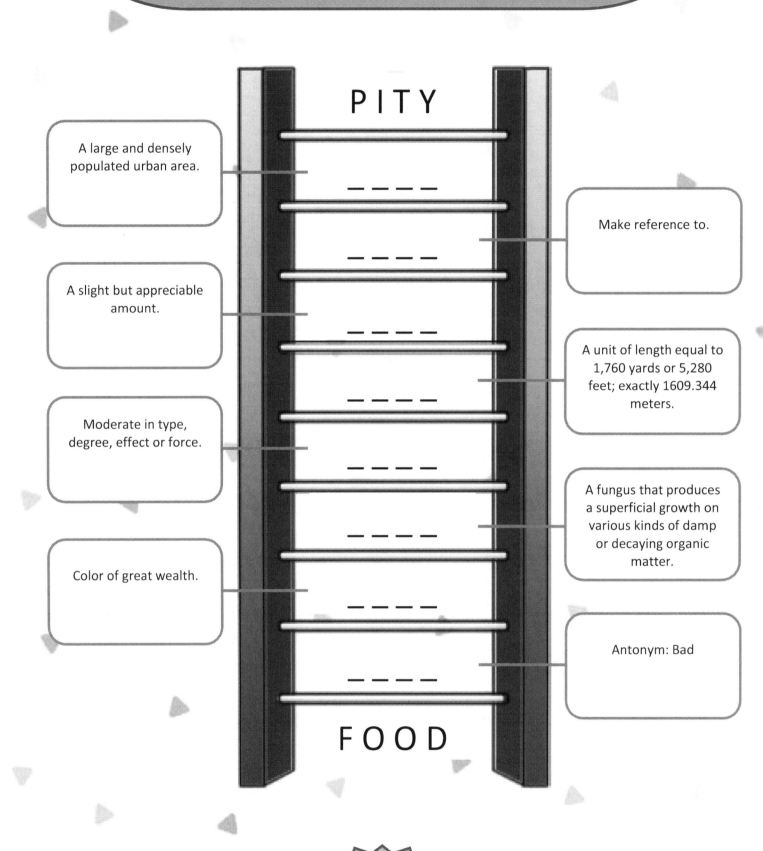

PITY

A large and densely populated urban area.

Make reference to.

A slight but appreciable amount.

A unit of length equal to 1,760 yards or 5,280 feet; exactly 1609.344 meters.

Moderate in type, degree, effect or force.

A fungus that produces a superficial growth on various kinds of damp or decaying organic matter.

Color of great wealth.

Antonym: Bad

FOOD

TREE

_ _ _ _

_ _ _

_ _ _ _

_ _ _ _

_ _ _ _

_ _ _ _

_ _ _ _

TALL

Costs nothing.

Something to walk on.

Knocked down.

A very large enclosed shopping area.

To worry.

Craft material made of matted fibers.

Another word for autumn.

High in stature.

FROM SEED TO DRAW

S E E D

Winter ride.

_ _ _ _

A whole bunch.

_ _ _ _

The opposite of fast.

_ _ _ _

Shine brightly.

_ _ _ _

Get bigger.

_ _ _ _

The part of the face above the eyes.

Drink made by steeping and boiling and fermenting rather than distilling.

_ _ _ _

_ _ _ _

Simple past tense form of the verb to draw.

D R A W

08

FROM GREEN TO BRASH

GREEN

Wanting everything.

Narrow-leaved green herbage.

Plant with trees.

Tall perennial woody plants having a main trunk and branches forming a distinct elevated crown.

A hairdo formed by braiding or twisting the hair.

Pungent leaves of any of numerous cruciferous herbs.

(Of persons) so unrefined as to be lacking in discrimination and sensibility.

An alloy of copper and zinc.

BRASH

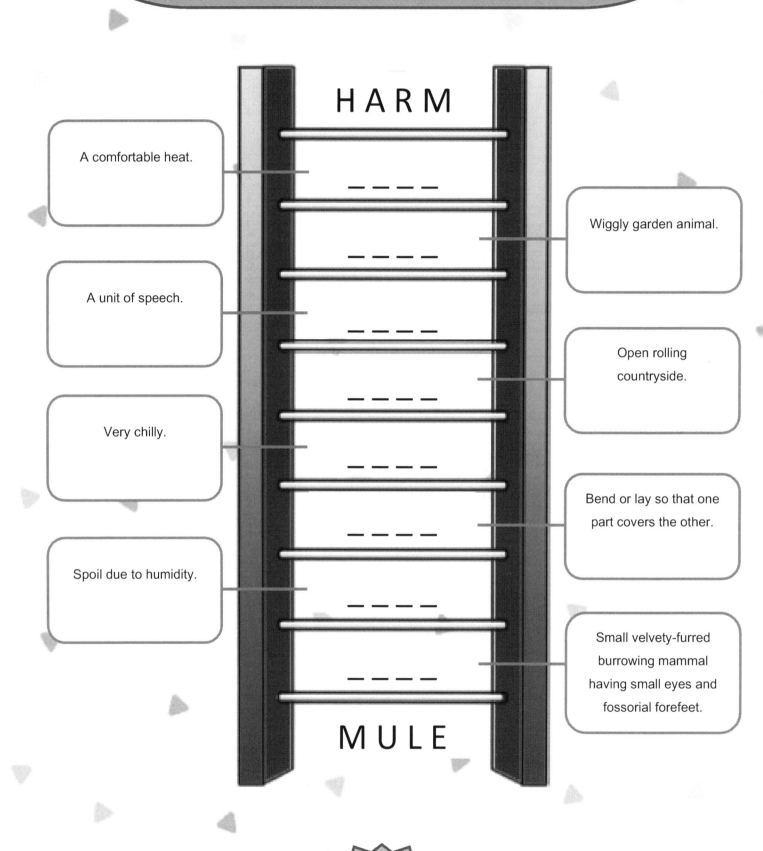

HARM

A comfortable heat.

_ _ _ _

Wiggly garden animal.

_ _ _ _

A unit of speech.

_ _ _ _

Open rolling countryside.

_ _ _ _

Very chilly.

_ _ _ _

Bend or lay so that one part covers the other.

Spoil due to humidity.

_ _ _ _

_ _ _ _

Small velvety-furred burrowing mammal having small eyes and fossorial forefeet.

MULE

FROM BELL TO BLUE

BELL

Exchange or deliver for money or its equivalent.

Acronym for Sea Air and Land.

_ _ _ _

Make very hot and dry.

_ _ _ _

A light in the night sky.

_ _ _ _

A part of training for a boxer.

_ _ _ _

Any sharply pointed projection.

_ _ _ _

A disparaging remark.

_ _ _ _

A hazy or indistinct representation.

_ _ _ _

BLUE

FROM TRIED TO FARTH

TRIED

Plural form of the noun trip.

Plural form of the noun grip.

Third-person singular form of the simple present indicative tense of the verb to grit.

Plural form of the noun writ.

Third-person singular form of the simple present indicative tense of the verb to wait.

Plural form of the noun wart.

Third-person singular form of the simple present indicative tense of the verb to fart.

Loyalty or allegiance to a cause or a person.

FAITH

HIDE

Large distance from side to side.

_ _ _ _

Grown-up drink.

_ _ _ _

Blowing air.

_ _ _ _

Discover.

That which is responsible for one's thoughts and feelings.

_ _ _ _

_ _ _ _

Moderate in type, degree, effect or force; far from extreme.

Machinery that processes materials by grinding or crushing.

_ _ _ _

_ _ _ _

A fixed and persistent intent or purpose.

WALL

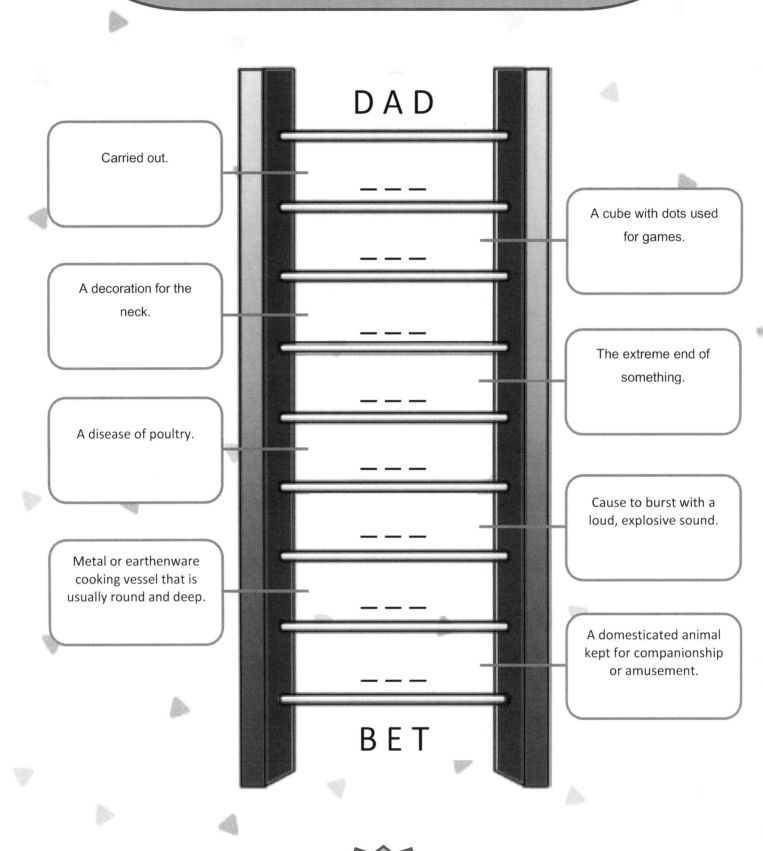

DAD

_ _ _

_ _ _

_ _ _

_ _ _

_ _ _

_ _ _

_ _ _

BET

Carried out.

A decoration for the neck.

A disease of poultry.

Metal or earthenware cooking vessel that is usually round and deep.

A cube with dots used for games.

The extreme end of something.

Cause to burst with a loud, explosive sound.

A domesticated animal kept for companionship or amusement.

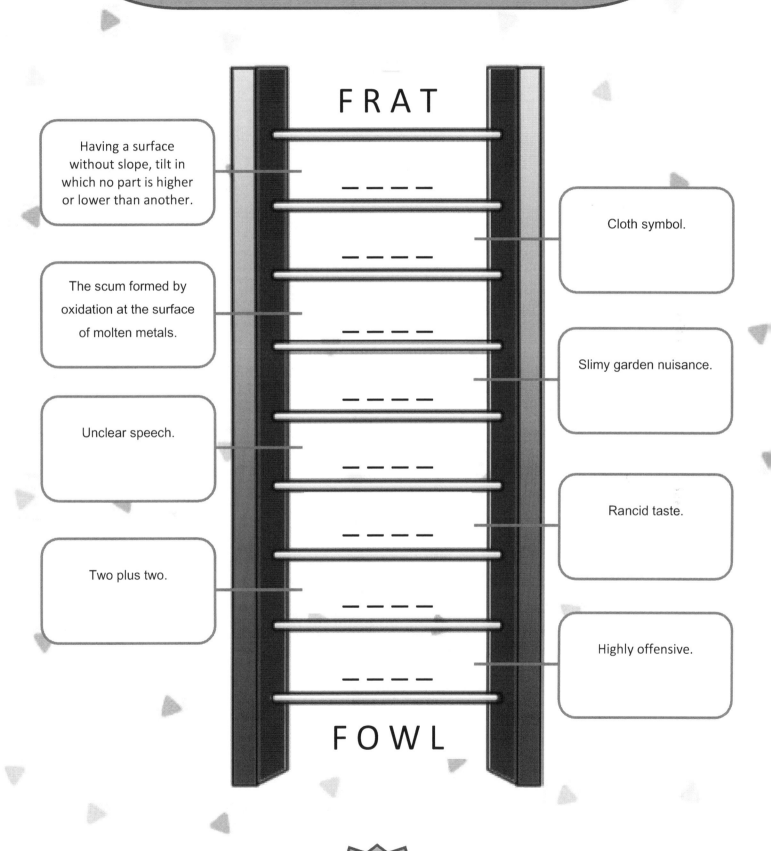

FRAT

Having a surface without slope, tilt in which no part is higher or lower than another.

Cloth symbol.

The scum formed by oxidation at the surface of molten metals.

Slimy garden nuisance.

Unclear speech.

Rancid taste.

Two plus two.

Highly offensive.

FOWL

FROM BATS TO BARE

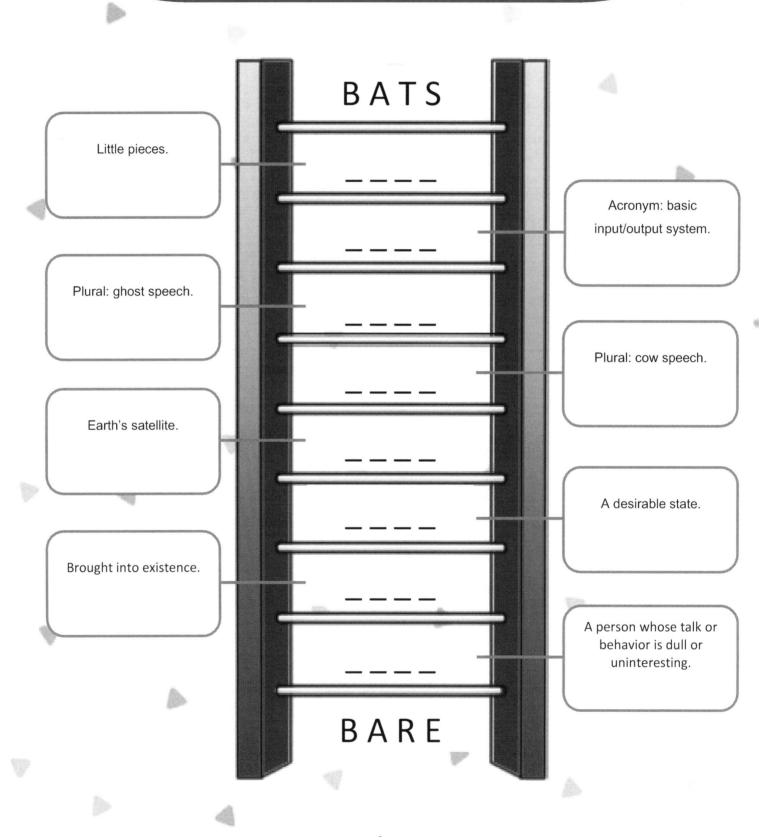

BATS

Little pieces.

_ _ _ _

Acronym: basic input/output system.

Plural: ghost speech.

_ _ _ _

Plural: cow speech.

Earth's satellite.

_ _ _ _

A desirable state.

Brought into existence.

_ _ _ _

A person whose talk or behavior is dull or uninteresting.

_ _ _ _

BARE

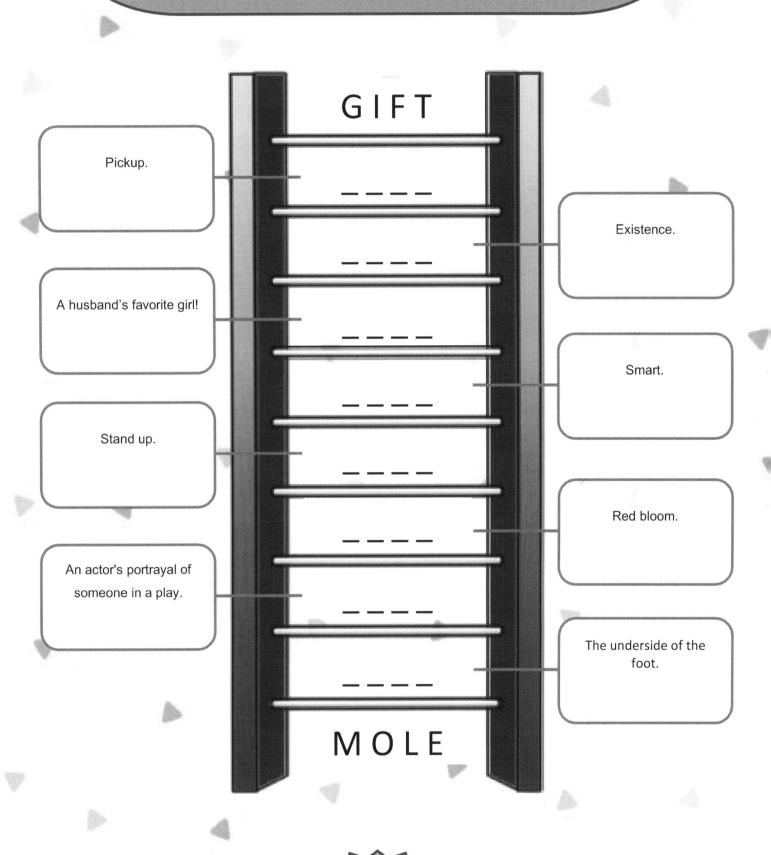

GIFT

_ _ _ _

_ _ _ _

_ _ _ _

_ _ _ _

_ _ _ _

_ _ _ _

_ _ _ _

MOLE

Pickup.

A husband's favorite girl!

Stand up.

An actor's portrayal of someone in a play.

Existence.

Smart.

Red bloom.

The underside of the foot.

TRAP

A four-wheeled wagon that runs on tracks in a mine.

_ _ _ _

A group with the same goal.

_ _ _ _

Fancy hardwood.

_ _ _ _

Top of a mountain.

_ _ _ _

To poke with a beak.

_ _ _ _

Rubber ice hockey disk.

_ _ _ _

Good fortune.

_ _ _ _

A piece of paper money worth one dollar.

_ _ _ _

BACK

LOOK

A written work or composition that has been published (printed on pages bound together).

_ _ _ _

Transform and make suitable for consumption by heating.

_ _ _ _

(Chess) the piece that can move any number of unoccupied squares in a direction parallel to the sides of the chessboard.

_ _ _ _

Representation of the cross on which Jesus died.

Any substance that can be metabolized by an animal to give energy and build tissue.

_ _ _ _

_ _ _ _

Having or displaying warmth or affection.

Try to manage without help.

_ _ _ _

_ _ _ _

Give temporarily; let have for a limited time.

_ _ _ _

MEND

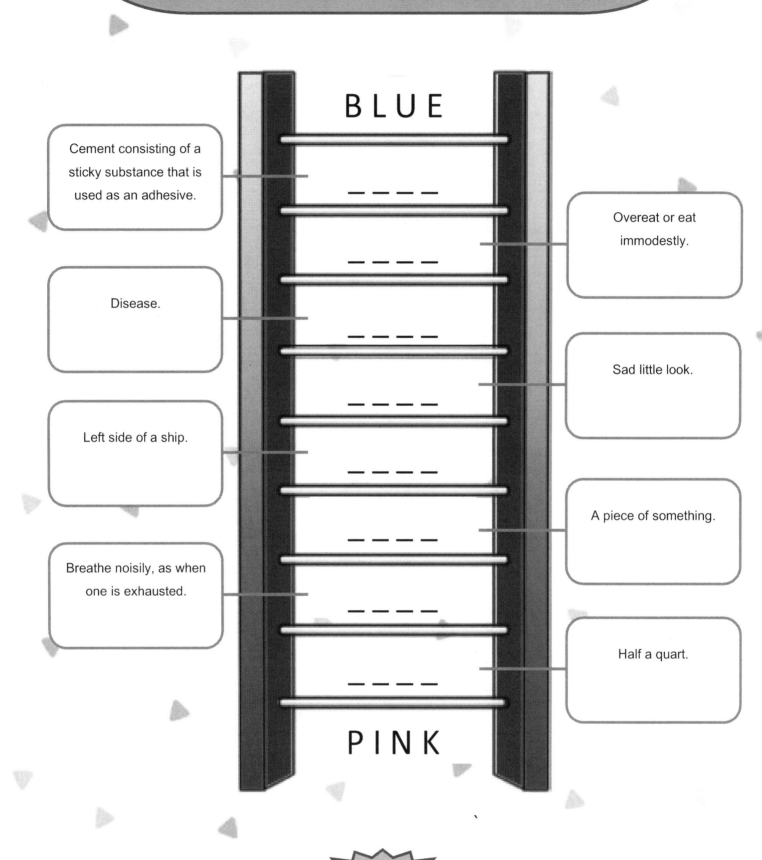

BLUE

Cement consisting of a sticky substance that is used as an adhesive.

Overeat or eat immodestly.

Disease.

Sad little look.

Left side of a ship.

A piece of something.

Breathe noisily, as when one is exhausted.

Half a quart.

PINK

FROM BEAL TO LOOK

BEAL

A blue-green color or pigment. ----

Genuine. ----

Interpret something that is written or printed. ----

A small ball with a hole through the middle. ----

To defeat someone in a race. ----

Floating vehicle. ----

Cowboy footwear. ----

Something to read. ----

LOOK

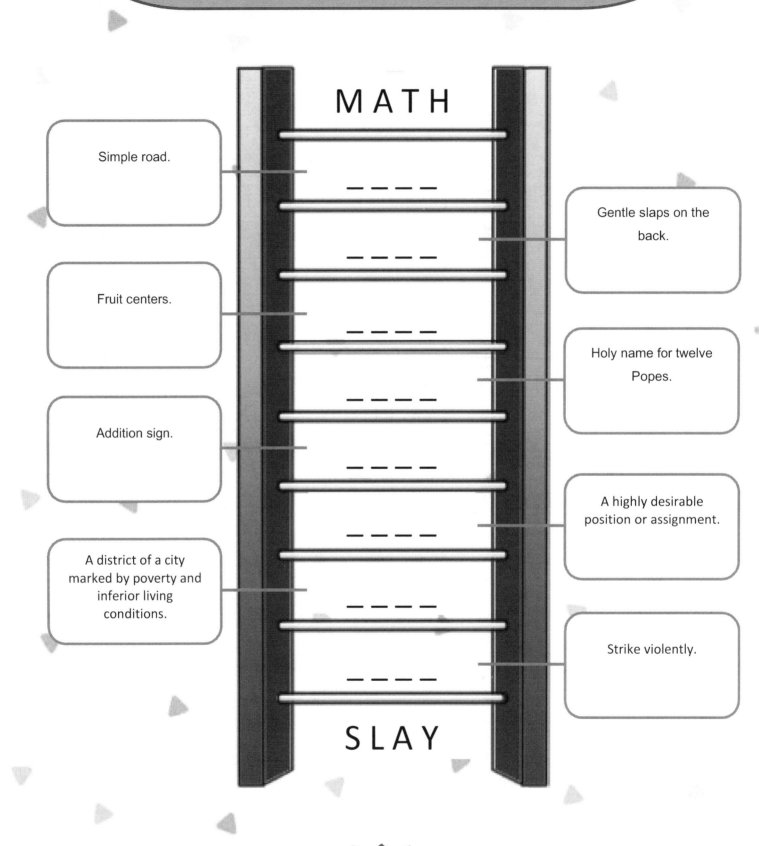

MATH

Simple road.

Gentle slaps on the back.

Fruit centers.

Holy name for twelve Popes.

Addition sign.

A highly desirable position or assignment.

A district of a city marked by poverty and inferior living conditions.

Strike violently.

SLAY

FROM WINK TO MITE

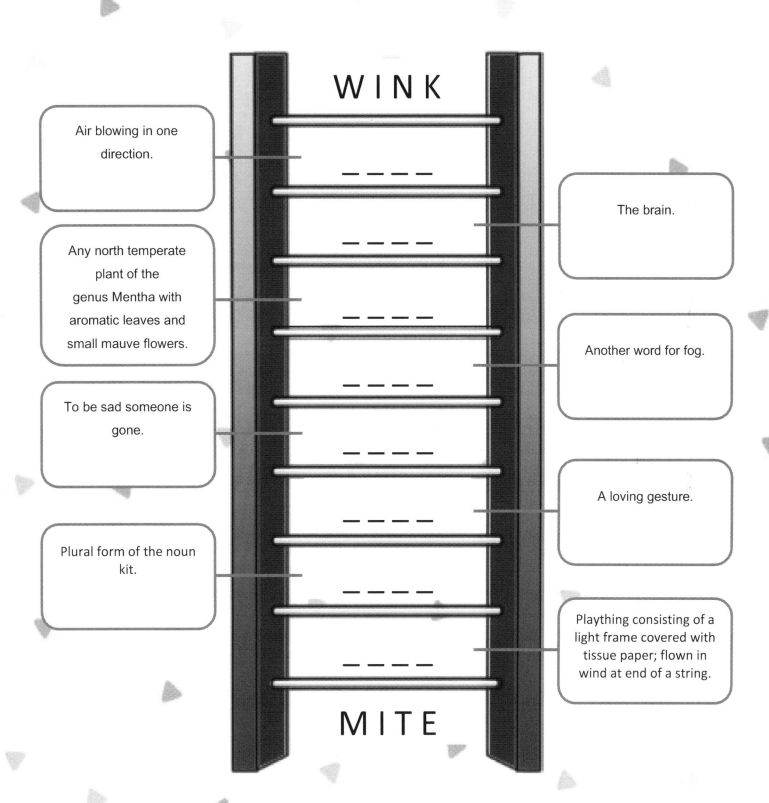

WINK

Air blowing in one direction.

_ _ _ _

The brain.

_ _ _ _

Any north temperate plant of the genus Mentha with aromatic leaves and small mauve flowers.

_ _ _ _

Another word for fog.

_ _ _ _

To be sad someone is gone.

_ _ _ _

A loving gesture.

_ _ _ _

Plural form of the noun kit.

_ _ _ _

Plaything consisting of a light frame covered with tissue paper; flown in wind at end of a string.

_ _ _ _

MITE

FROM SMILE TO TEARS

SMILE

Inflict a heavy blow on, with the hand, a tool, or a weapon.

Speaking of oneself in a positive way with too much pride or self-indulgence.

Sports equipment that is worn on the feet to enable the wearer to glide along and to be propelled by the alternate actions of the legs.

Thin layers of rock used for roofing.

Disposed to avoid notice.

Third-person singular form of the simple present indicative tense of the verb to blat.

Third-person singular form of the simple present indicative tense of the verb to beat.

Large mammals with long shaggy coat and strong claws.

TEARS

FROM SKIP TO SEED

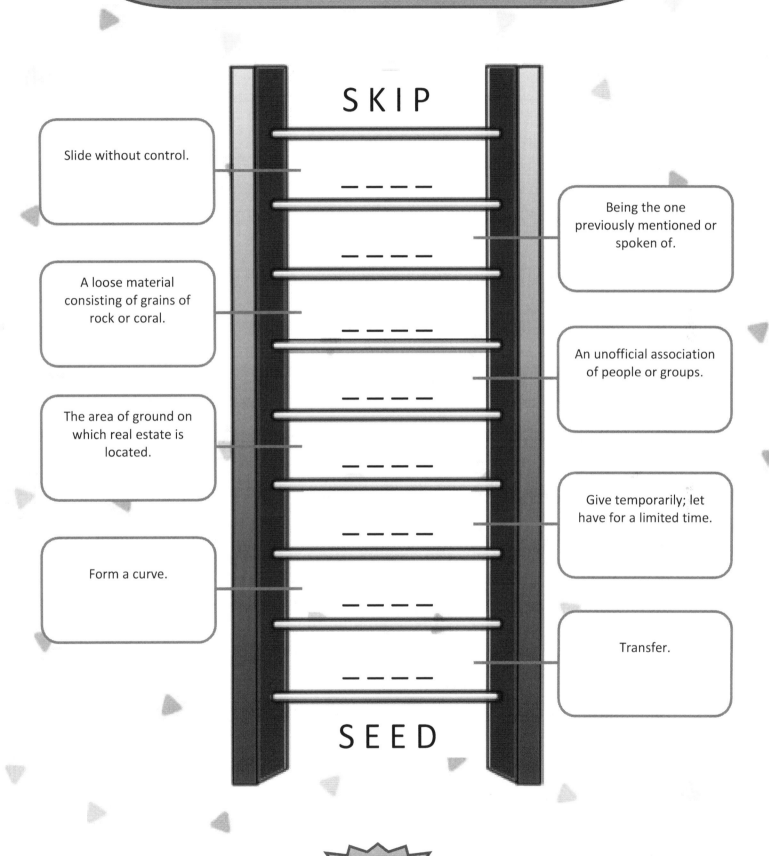

SKIP

Slide without control.

Being the one previously mentioned or spoken of.

A loose material consisting of grains of rock or coral.

An unofficial association of people or groups.

The area of ground on which real estate is located.

Give temporarily; let have for a limited time.

Form a curve.

Transfer.

SEED

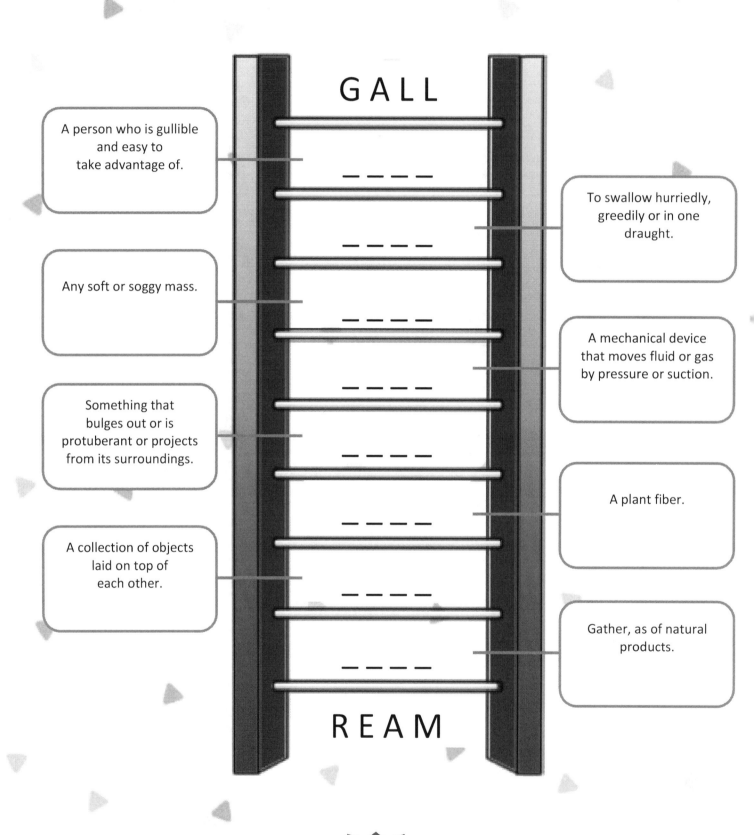

GALL

A person who is gullible and easy to take advantage of.

To swallow hurriedly, greedily or in one draught.

Any soft or soggy mass.

A mechanical device that moves fluid or gas by pressure or suction.

Something that bulges out or is protuberant or projects from its surroundings.

A plant fiber.

A collection of objects laid on top of each other.

Gather, as of natural products.

REAM

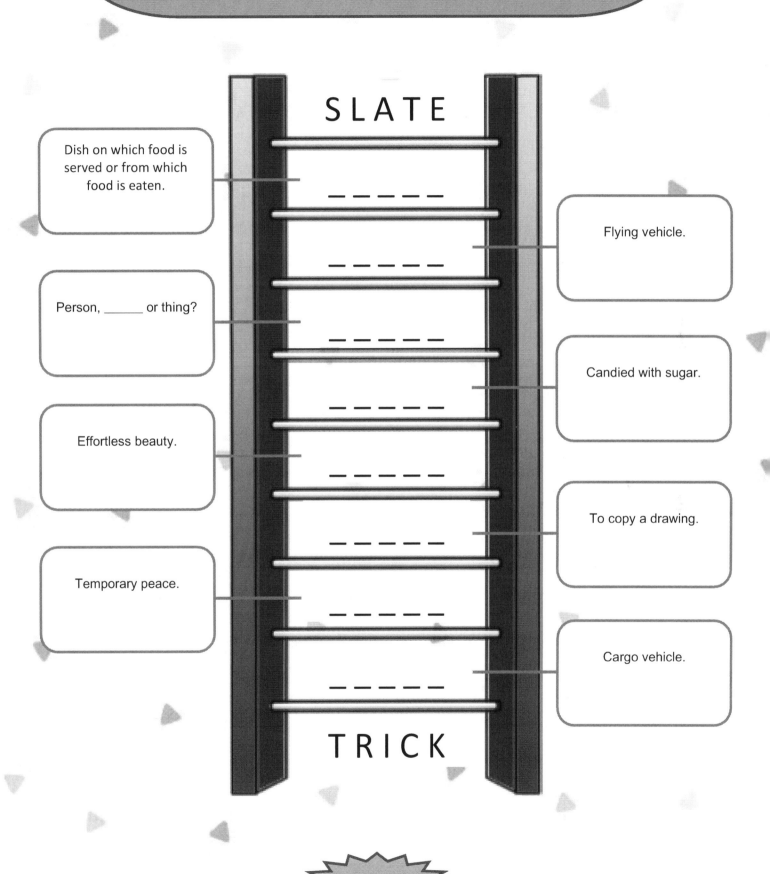

SLATE

Dish on which food is served or from which food is eaten.

Flying vehicle.

Person, _____ or thing?

Candied with sugar.

Effortless beauty.

To copy a drawing.

Temporary peace.

Cargo vehicle.

TRICK

FROM RAIN TO DINE

RAIN

Search without warning.

Spoke in the past.

_ _ _ _

Finely broken rock.

_ _ _ _

Magical stick.

Blowing air

_ _ _ _

_ _ _ _

Make a discovery.

Being satisfactory or in satisfactory condition

_ _ _ _

_ _ _ _

Belonging to me.

_ _ _ _

DINE

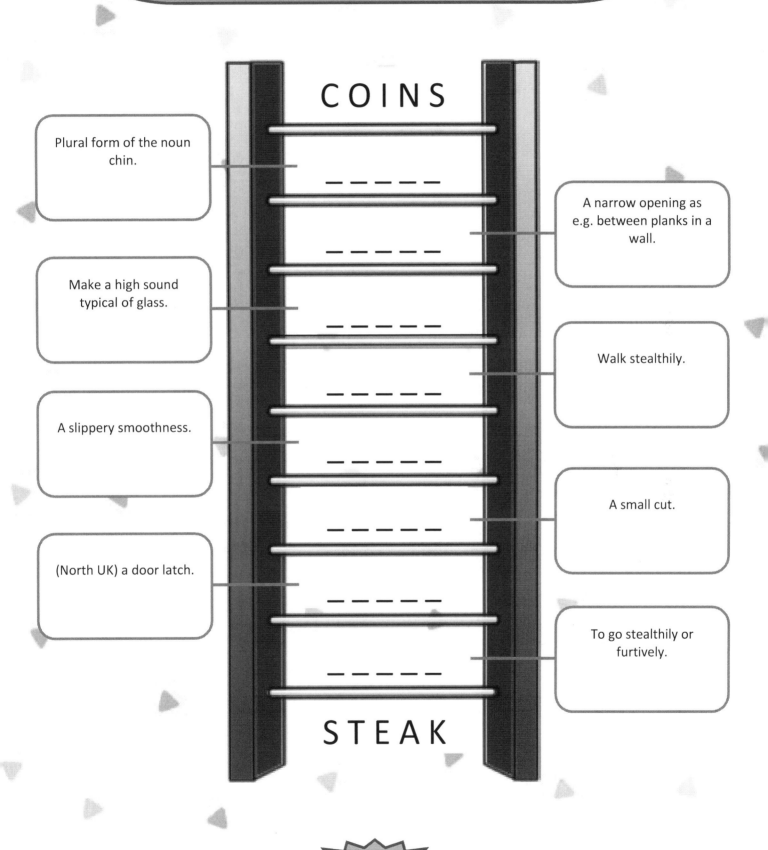

COINS

Plural form of the noun chin.

A narrow opening as e.g. between planks in a wall.

Make a high sound typical of glass.

Walk stealthily.

A slippery smoothness.

A small cut.

(North UK) a door latch.

To go stealthily or furtively.

STEAK

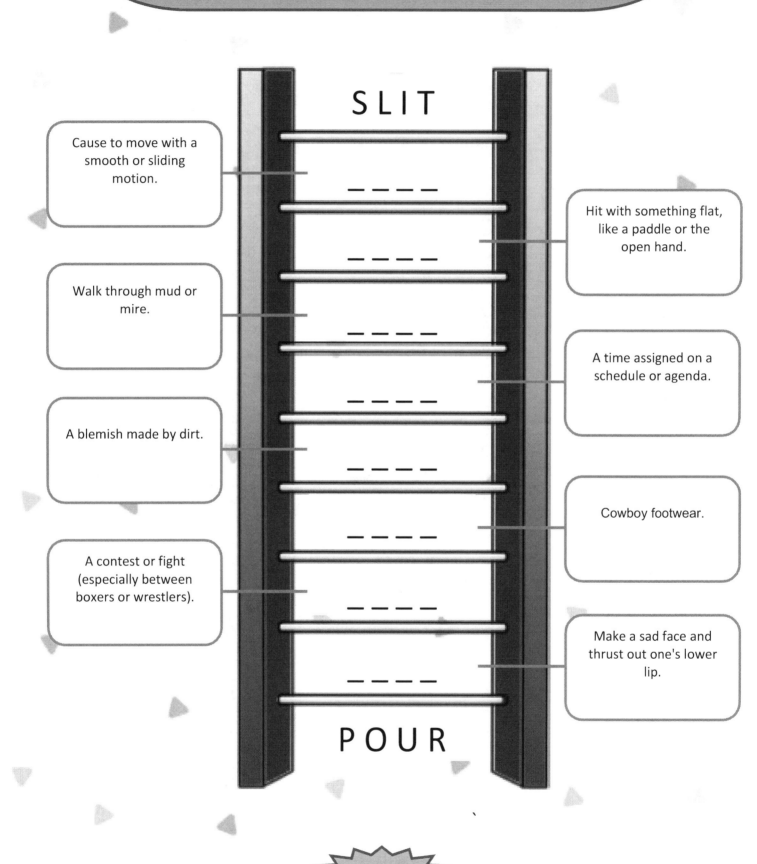

SLIT

Cause to move with a smooth or sliding motion.

_ _ _ _

Hit with something flat, like a paddle or the open hand.

_ _ _ _

Walk through mud or mire.

_ _ _ _

A time assigned on a schedule or agenda.

_ _ _ _

A blemish made by dirt.

_ _ _ _

Cowboy footwear.

_ _ _ _

A contest or fight (especially between boxers or wrestlers).

_ _ _ _

Make a sad face and thrust out one's lower lip.

_ _ _ _

POUR

HOLD

Simple past tense form of the verb to hoe.

_ _ _ _

Pay close attention to.

_ _ _ _

The upper part of the human body or the front part of the body in animals..

_ _ _ _

A collection of objects laid on top of each other.

_ _ _ _

Gather, as of natural products.

_ _ _ _

The part of something that is furthest from the normal viewer.

_ _ _ _

Large mammal with long shaggy coat and strong claws.

_ _ _ _

To separate or be separated by force.

_ _ _ _

TEAM

MATE

_ _ _ _

_ _ _ _

_ _ _ _

_ _ _ _

_ _ _ _

_ _ _ _

_ _ _ _

COSY

Moderate or restrain; lessen the force of.

A narrow thin strip of wood used as backing for plaster or to make latticework.

Function as a laser.

(Art) assume a posture as for artistic purposes.

Later than usual or than expected.

Beat severely with a whip or rod.

Fail to win.

An arrangement of flowers that is usually given as a present.

FROM PLOT TO DRAW

PLOT

A small slit (as for inserting a coin or depositing mail) — _ _ _ _

A blemish made by dirt — _ _ _ _

A group of countries in special alliance — _ _ _ _

A powerful stroke with the fist or a weapon — _ _ _ _

Shine intensely, as if with heat — _ _ _ _

Increase in size by natural process. — _ _ _ _

Simple past tense form of the verb to grow. — _ _ _ _

Simple past tense form of the verb to draw. — _ _ _ _

DRAW

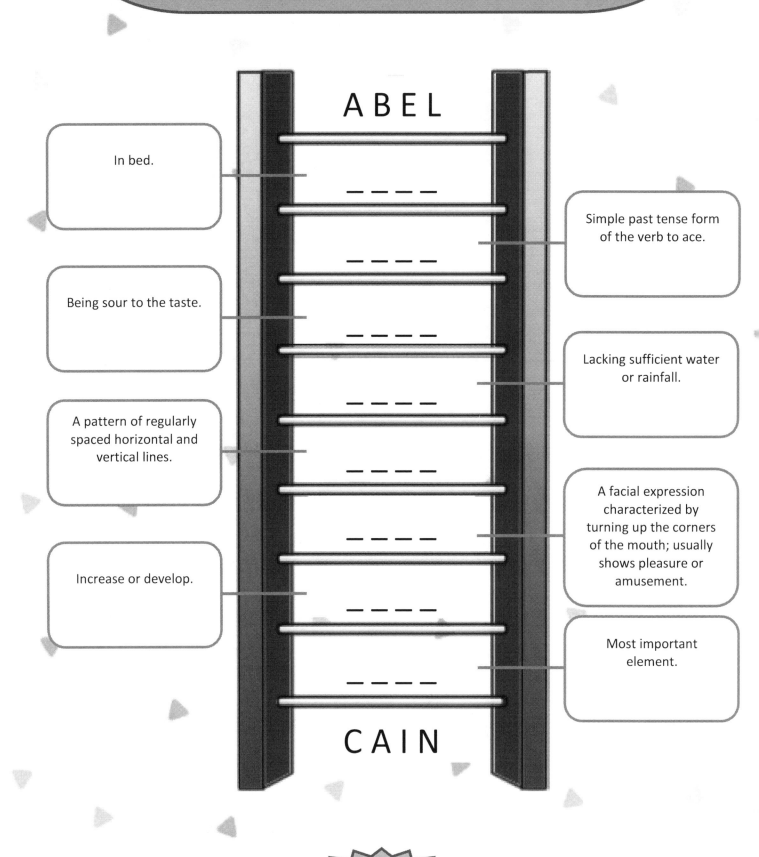

ABEL

In bed.

_ _ _ _

Simple past tense form of the verb to ace.

_ _ _ _

Being sour to the taste.

_ _ _ _

Lacking sufficient water or rainfall.

_ _ _ _

A pattern of regularly spaced horizontal and vertical lines.

_ _ _ _

A facial expression characterized by turning up the corners of the mouth; usually shows pleasure or amusement.

_ _ _ _

Increase or develop.

_ _ _ _

Most important element.

_ _ _ _

CAIN

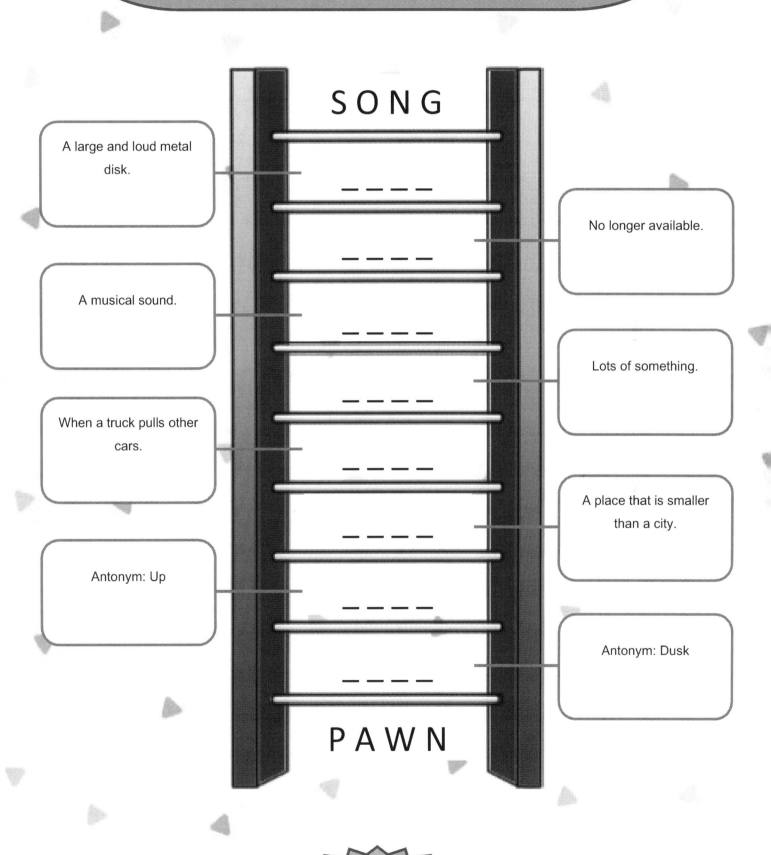

SONG

A large and loud metal disk.

No longer available.

_ _ _ _

A musical sound.

_ _ _ _

Lots of something.

_ _ _ _

When a truck pulls other cars.

_ _ _ _

A place that is smaller than a city.

_ _ _ _

Antonym: Up

_ _ _ _

Antonym: Dusk

_ _ _ _

PAWN

FROM BEAST TO VOGIE

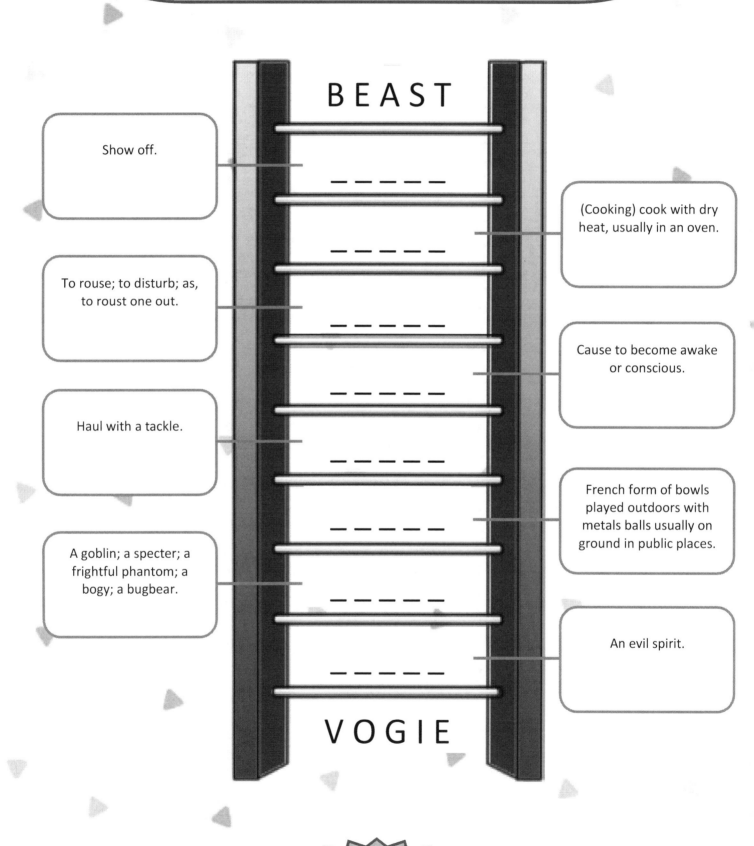

BEAST

Show off.

(Cooking) cook with dry heat, usually in an oven.

To rouse; to disturb; as, to roust one out.

Cause to become awake or conscious.

Haul with a tackle.

French form of bowls played outdoors with metals balls usually on ground in public places.

A goblin; a specter; a frightful phantom; a bogy; a bugbear.

An evil spirit.

VOGIE

FROM DRAY TO SLOW

DRAY

Make a mark or lines on a surface.

Simple past tense form of the verb to draw.

_ _ _ _

Simple past tense form of the verb to grow.

Become larger, greater, or bigger; expand or gain.

_ _ _ _

Shine intensely, as if with heat

_ _ _ _

A powerful stroke with the fist or a weapon

_ _ _ _

A shared on-line journal where people can post daily entries about their personal experiences and hobbies.

_ _ _ _

Work doggedly or persistently.

_ _ _ _

SLOW

FROM NAVY TO ARTY

NAVY

(Used with singular count nouns) colloquial for 'not a' or 'not one' or 'never a'.

The mother of Jesus; Christians refer to her as the Virgin Mary; she is especially honored by Roman Catholics.

_ _ _ _

(Of soil) soft and watery.

_ _ _ _

Open to or abounding in fresh air.

Affected manners intended to impress others.

_ _ _ _

Third-person singular form of the simple present indicative tense of the verb to aim.

_ _ _ _

Weapons considered collectively.

_ _ _ _

(Military) a permanent organization of the military land forces of a nation or state.

ARTY

FROM SHELF TO STACK

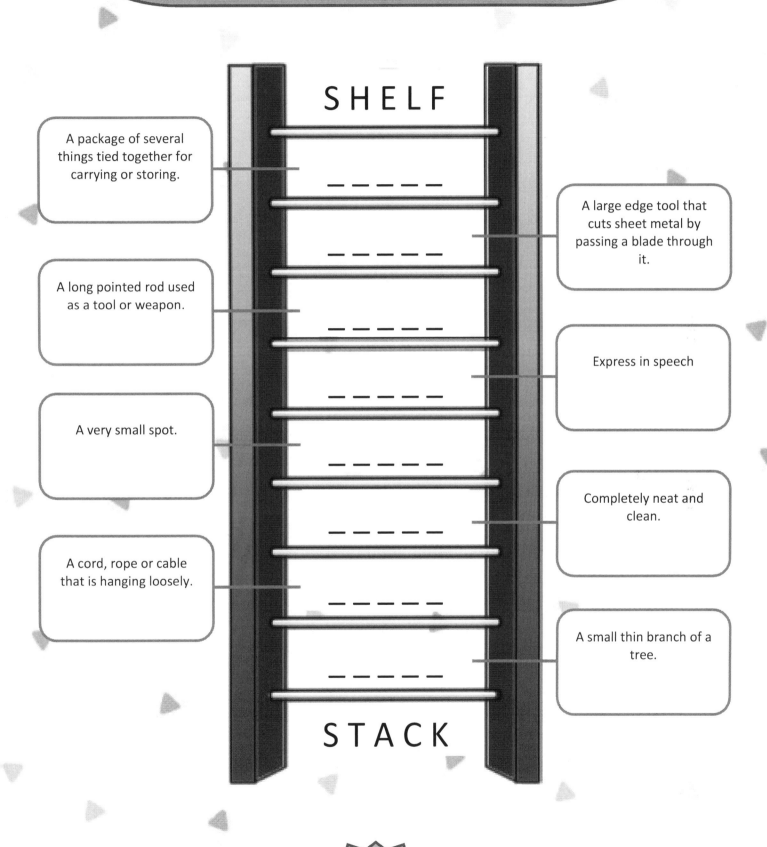

SHELF

A package of several things tied together for carrying or storing.

A large edge tool that cuts sheet metal by passing a blade through it.

A long pointed rod used as a tool or weapon.

Express in speech

A very small spot.

Completely neat and clean.

A cord, rope or cable that is hanging loosely.

A small thin branch of a tree.

STACK

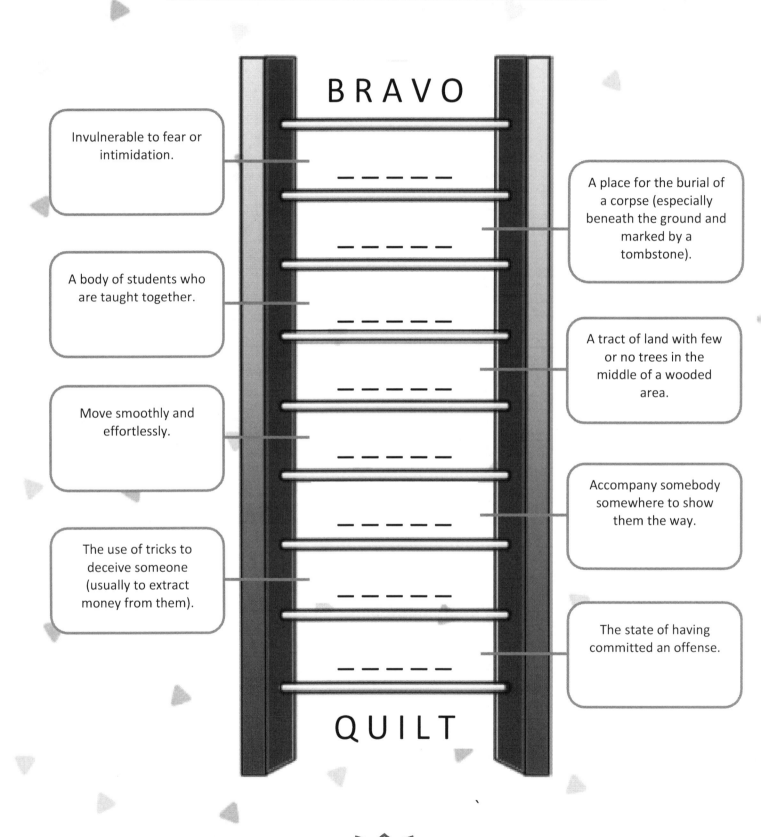

BRAVO

Invulnerable to fear or intimidation.

A place for the burial of a corpse (especially beneath the ground and marked by a tombstone).

A body of students who are taught together.

A tract of land with few or no trees in the middle of a wooded area.

Move smoothly and effortlessly.

Accompany somebody somewhere to show them the way.

The use of tricks to deceive someone (usually to extract money from them).

The state of having committed an offense.

QUILT

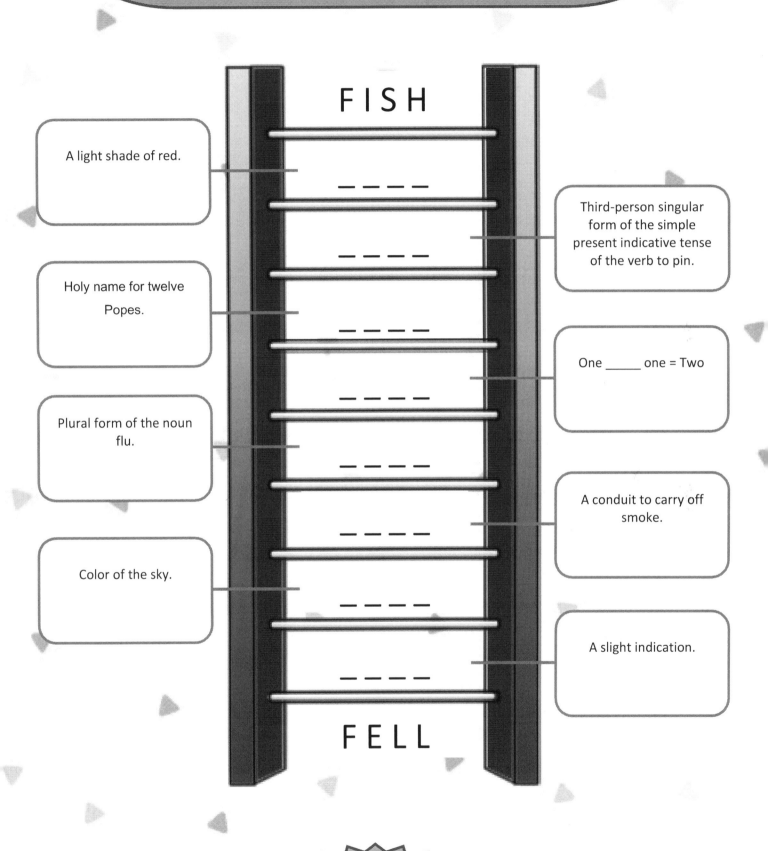

FISH

_ _ _ _

_ _ _ _

_ _ _ _

_ _ _ _

_ _ _ _

_ _ _ _

_ _ _ _

FELL

A light shade of red.

Holy name for twelve Popes.

Plural form of the noun flu.

Color of the sky.

Third-person singular form of the simple present indicative tense of the verb to pin.

One _____ one = Two

A conduit to carry off smoke.

A slight indication.

CRUST

The top line of a hill, mountain, or wave.

_ _ _ _ _

A port city in northwestern France (in Brittany); the chief naval station of France.

Highly favored or fortunate (as e.g. by divine grace).

_ _ _ _ _

Simple past tense and past participle of blend.

Used of a knife or other blade; not sharp.

_ _ _ _ _

A name given to several different species of plants having blue flowers.

A state of depression.

_ _ _ _ _

Plural form of the noun flue.

_ _ _ _ _

FLIES

KETTLE

Take up residence and become established.

_ _ _ _ _ _

A small sofa.

One who sets written material into type.

_ _ _ _ _ _

Comparative form: good.

A liquid or semiliquid mixture, as of flour, eggs, and milk, used in cooking.

_ _ _ _ _ _

_ _ _ _ _ _

Comparative form: fat.

Be unsure or weak.

_ _ _ _ _ _

Device that removes something from whatever passes through it.

_ _ _ _ _ _

FILLER

FROM WINTER to SUMMER

WINTER

A worker who winds (e.g., a winch, clock or other mechanism).

_ _ _ _ _ _

Move about aimlessly or without any destination, often in search of food or employment.

A person who works in a prison and is in charge of prisoners.

_ _ _ _ _ _

Antonym: Easier.

Someone who plays the harp.

_ _ _ _ _ _

A basket usually with a cover.

A hand tool with a heavy rigid head and a handle.

_ _ _ _ _ _

A singer who produces a tune without opening the lips or forming words.

SUMMER

FROM ROUGE TO CHOCK

ROUGE

An established line of travel or access.

Overwhelming defeats.

_ _ _ _ _

The condition of belonging to a particular place or group by virtue of social or ethnic or cultural lineage.

_ _ _ _ _

Plural form of the noun boot.

_ _ _ _ _

Blemishes made by dirt.

_ _ _ _ _

Plural form of the noun bloc.

_ _ _ _ _

A solid piece of something (usually having flat rectangular sides).

_ _ _ _ _

A timepiece that shows the time of day.

_ _ _ _ _

CHOCK

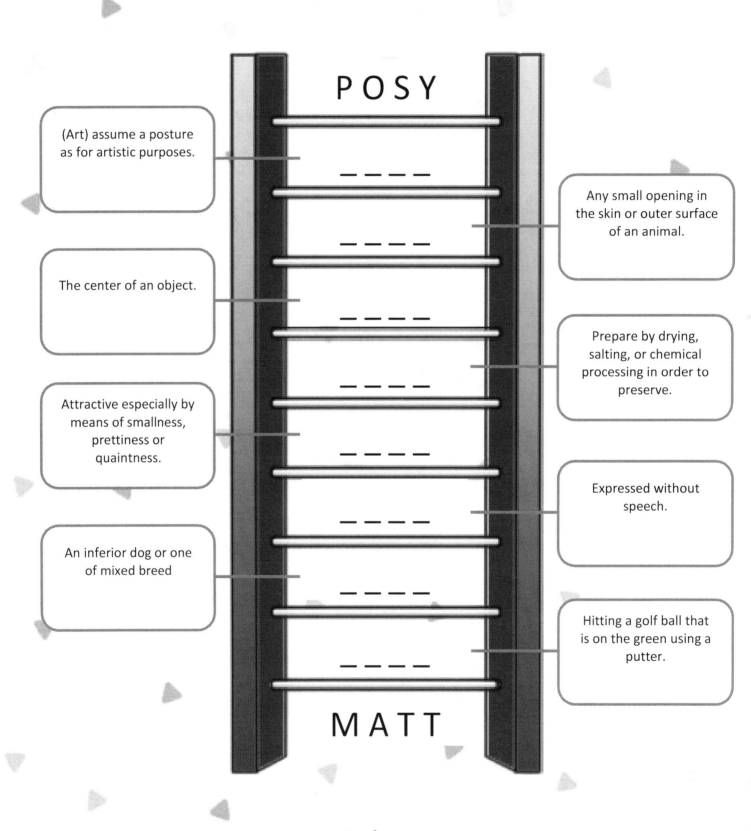

POSY

(Art) assume a posture as for artistic purposes.

Any small opening in the skin or outer surface of an animal.

The center of an object.

Prepare by drying, salting, or chemical processing in order to preserve.

Attractive especially by means of smallness, prettiness or quaintness.

Expressed without speech.

An inferior dog or one of mixed breed

Hitting a golf ball that is on the green using a putter.

MATT

FROM GUNS TO LUTE

GUNS

_ _ _ _

_ _ _ _

_ _ _ _

_ _ _ _

_ _ _ _

_ _ _ _

_ _ _ _

LUTE

Plural form of the noun gin.

Plural form of the noun bit.

A valley.

The specified day of the month.

Plural form of the noun bin.

A small amount of solid food; a mouthful.

An event (or a course of events) that will inevitably happen in the future.

Later than usual or than expected.

SALE

Antonym: Different.

_ _ _ _

Mentally healthy; free from mental disorder.

_ _ _ _

Grow smaller.

_ _ _ _

Hunt or look for; require for a particular reason.

_ _ _ _

Breathe noisily, as when one is exhausted.

_ _ _ _

Sheet glass cut in shapes for windows or doors.

_ _ _ _

Very light colored; highly diluted with white.

_ _ _ _

Characteristic of a man.

_ _ _ _

MULE

FROM LANE TO MUCH

LANE

_ _ _ _

_ _ _ _

_ _ _ _

_ _ _ _

_ _ _ _

_ _ _ _

_ _ _ _

MUCH

Long coarse hair growing from the crest of the animal's neck.

One; single.

Treat with contempt.

Draw into the mouth by creating a practical vacuum in the mouth.

The muller, or crushing and grinding stone.

A male religious living in a cloister and devoting himself to contemplation and prayer and work.

Worn inside the shoe.

To so extreme a degree.

ROUTS

Plural form of the noun root.

Plural form of the noun coot.

Plural form of the noun coon.

_ _ _ _ _

Plural form of the noun coin.

Plural form of the noun chin.

_ _ _ _ _

A narrow opening as e.g. between planks in a wall

Informal term for a (young) woman.

_ _ _ _ _

Examine so as to determine accuracy, quality, or condition.

CHECK

TURF

Waves breaking on the shore.

(Middle Ages) a person who is bound to the land and owned by the feudal lord.

_ _ _ _

Your consciousness of your own identity.

Exchange or deliver for money or its equivalent.

_ _ _ _

(Geology) a flat (usually horizontal) mass of igneous rock between two layers of older sedimentary rock.

_ _ _ _

Any of various young herrings (other than brislings) canned as sardines in Norway.

_ _ _ _

A region of southeastern Pakistan.

_ _ _ _

Transfer.

_ _ _ _

TEND

FROM DATE TO AWED

DATE

(Chess) place an opponent's king under an attack from which it cannot escape and thus ending the game.

Plural form of the noun mat.

Plural form of the noun oat.

Plural form of the noun ort.

Plural form of the noun orb.

Plural form of the noun ore.

Third-person singular form of the simple present indicative tense of the verb to owe.

Simple past tense form of the verb to owe.

AWED

STAR

A part of training for a boxer.

_ _ _ _

To cover or extend over an area or time period.

Revolve quickly and repeatedly around one's own axis.

_ _ _ _

Expel or eject (saliva or phlegm or sputum) from the mouth.

_ _ _ _

A set of garments (usually including a jacket and trousers or skirt) for outerwear all of the same fabric and

_ _ _ _

Put an end to a state or an activity.

[UK] The basic unit of money in Great Britain and Northern Ireland; equal to 100 pence.

_ _ _ _

One of five children born at the same time from the same pregnancy.

_ _ _ _

RUIN

LEWD

Accompany somebody somewhere to show them the way.

`_ _ _ _`

Weight to be borne or conveyed.

`_ _ _ _`

A rich soil consisting of a mixture of sand and clay and decaying organic materials.

`_ _ _ _`

Move about aimlessly or without any destination, often in search of food or employment.

`_ _ _ _`

Utter words loudly and forcefully.

`_ _ _ _`

An uncastrated male hog.

A small vessel for travel on water.

`_ _ _ _`

A discharge of lightning accompanied by thunder.

`_ _ _ _`

HOLT

FROM PUMP TO BARE

PUMP

_ _ _ _

_ _ _ _

_ _ _ _

_ _ _ _

_ _ _ _

_ _ _ _

_ _ _ _

BARE

A large bundle bound for storage or transport

A movable staircase that passengers use to board or leave an aircraft.

1. Plural form of the noun rat.

Flap the wings wildly or frantically; used of falcons.

Play boisterously.

1. Plural form of the noun ram.

Amount of a charge or payment relative to some basis.

A large bundle bound for storage or transport.

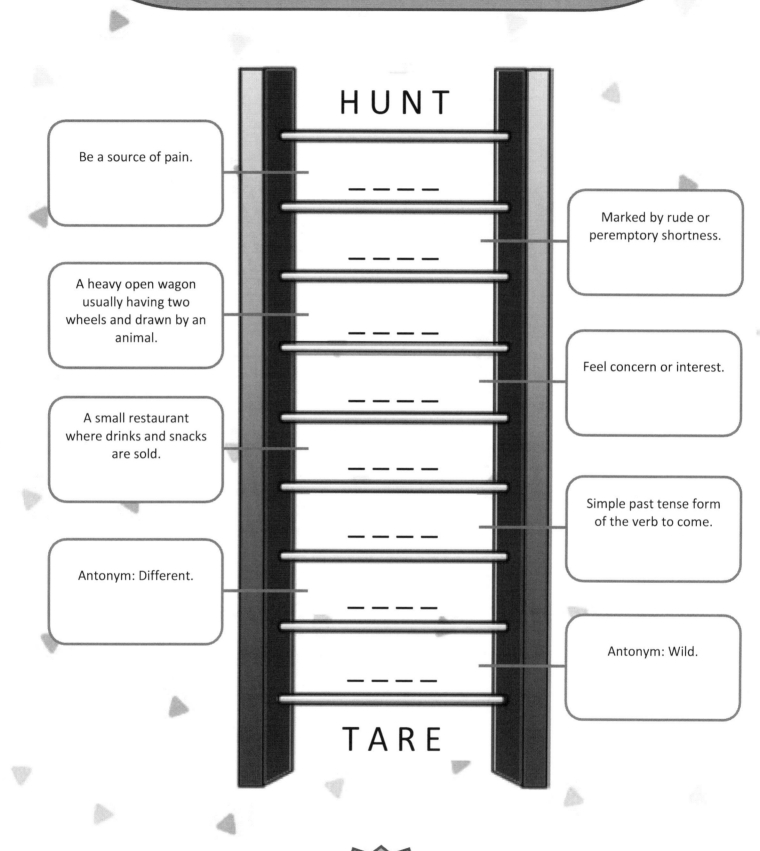

HUNT

Be a source of pain.

Marked by rude or peremptory shortness.

A heavy open wagon usually having two wheels and drawn by an animal.

Feel concern or interest.

A small restaurant where drinks and snacks are sold.

Simple past tense form of the verb to come.

Antonym: Different.

Antonym: Wild.

TARE

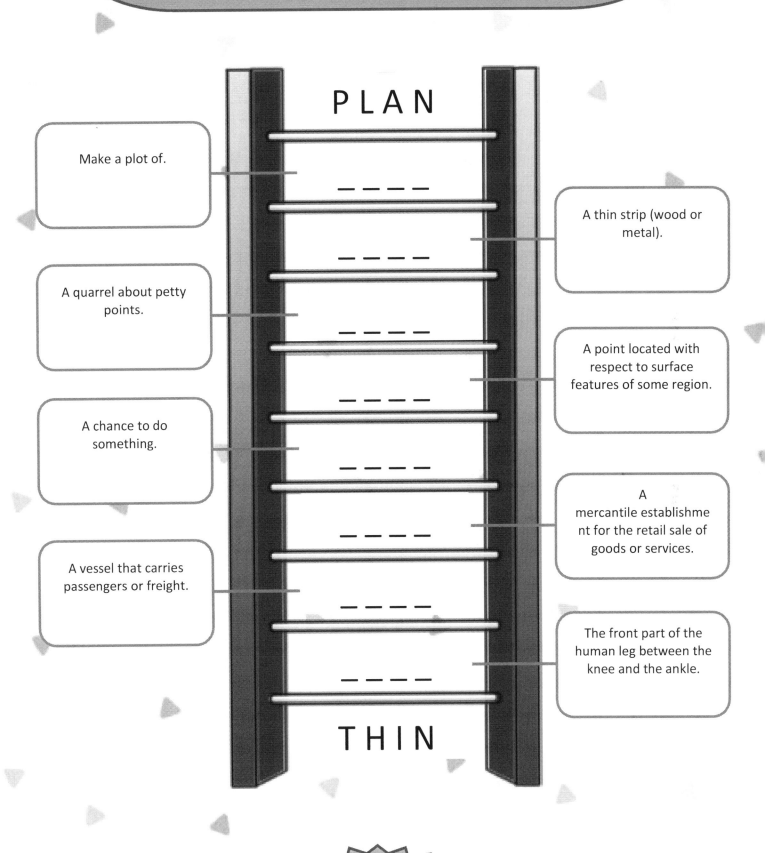

PLAN

Make a plot of.

A thin strip (wood or metal).

_ _ _ _

A quarrel about petty points.

_ _ _ _

_ _ _ _

A point located with respect to surface features of some region.

A chance to do something.

_ _ _ _

A mercantile establishme nt for the retail sale of goods or services.

A vessel that carries passengers or freight.

_ _ _ _

_ _ _ _

The front part of the human leg between the knee and the ankle.

_ _ _ _

THIN

CUED

The thick white substance which is formed when milk turns sour.

_ _ _ _

A line made of twisted fibers or threads.

_ _ _ _

A brief statement.

_ _ _ _

The hard fibrous lignified substance under the bark of trees.

_ _ _ _

A fabric made from the hair of sheep.

_ _ _ _

An excavation that is (usually) filled with water.

_ _ _ _

A person who lacks good judgment.

_ _ _ _

Violating accepted standards or rules.

_ _ _ _

SOUL

58

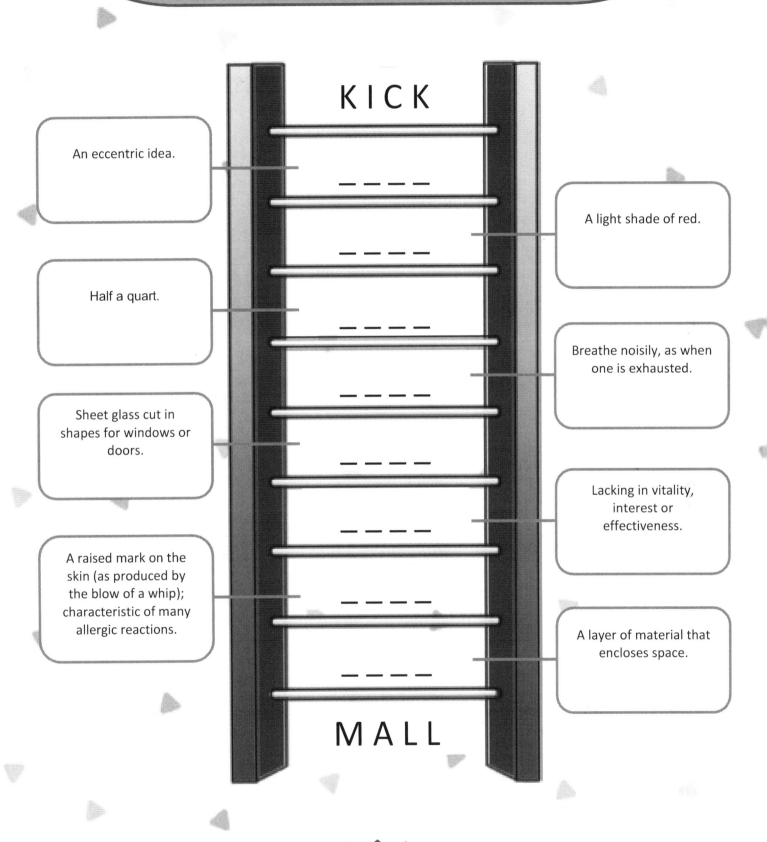

KICK

An eccentric idea.

A light shade of red.

Half a quart.

Breathe noisily, as when one is exhausted.

Sheet glass cut in shapes for windows or doors.

Lacking in vitality, interest or effectiveness.

A raised mark on the skin (as produced by the blow of a whip); characteristic of many allergic reactions.

A layer of material that encloses space.

MALL

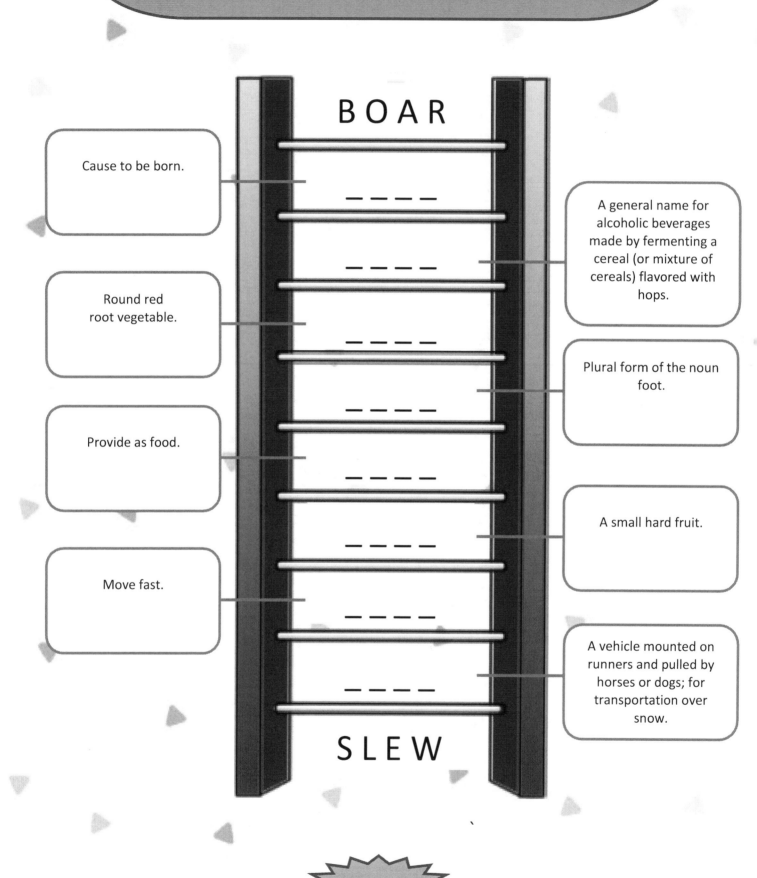

BOAR

Cause to be born.

A general name for alcoholic beverages made by fermenting a cereal (or mixture of cereals) flavored with hops.

Round red root vegetable.

Plural form of the noun foot.

Provide as food.

A small hard fruit.

Move fast.

A vehicle mounted on runners and pulled by horses or dogs; for transportation over snow.

SLEW

FROM LURK TO CURE

LURK

_ _ _ _

_ _ _ _

_ _ _ _

_ _ _ _

_ _ _ _

_ _ _ _

_ _ _ _

_ _ _ _

CURE

Make dark, dim, or gloomy.

A covering to disguise or conceal the face.

Not reflecting light; not glossy.

Expressed without speech.

Used as a perfume fixative.

A vertical spar for supporting sails.

An inferior dog or one of mixed breed.

Attractive especially by means of smallness, prettiness or quaintness.

FROM REAR TO MOOD

REAR

_ _ _ _

A large quantity of written matter.

A gymnastic apparatus used by women gymnasts.

_ _ _ _

A cooperative unit (especially in sports).

_ _ _ _

Move in large numbers.

_ _ _ _

Simple past tense form of the verb to tee.

_ _ _ _

Having a toe or toes of a specified kind; often used in combination.

_ _ _ _

Simple past tense form of the verb to hoe.

_ _ _ _

A headdress that protects the head and face.

_ _ _ _

MOOD

FROM LOAF TO FEET

LOAF

The main organ of photosynthesis and transpiration in higher plants.

_ _ _ _

An artificial water trench, esp. one to or from a mill.

An accidental hole that allows something (fluid or light etc.) to enter or escape.

_ _ _ _

The most extreme possible amount or value.

A secret look.

_ _ _ _

Smell badly and offensively.

Related to onions; white cylindrical bulb and flat dark-green leaves.

_ _ _ _

[UK] A portion or list, especially a list of candidates for an office.

_ _ _ _

FEET

FROM LUNE TO GAPE

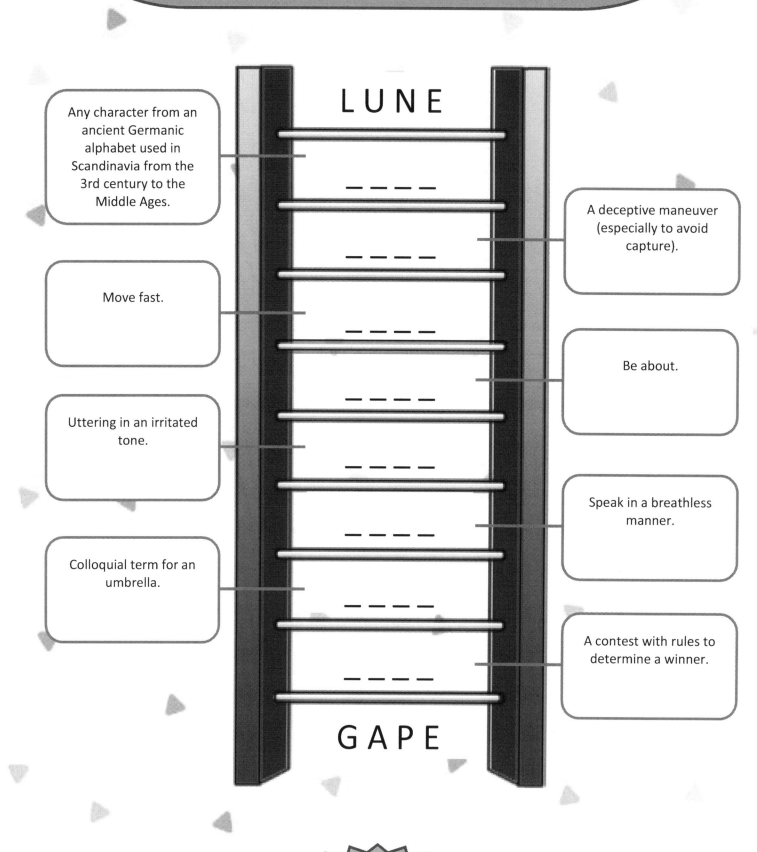

LUNE

Any character from an ancient Germanic alphabet used in Scandinavia from the 3rd century to the Middle Ages.

A deceptive maneuver (especially to avoid capture).

Move fast.

Be about.

Uttering in an irritated tone.

Speak in a breathless manner.

Colloquial term for an umbrella.

A contest with rules to determine a winner.

GAPE

FROM TORT TO FACE

TORT

A sheltered area of coast where ships can dock or anchor safely.

A written agreement between two states or sovereigns.

A mischievous sprite of English folklore.

The state of needing something that is absent or unavailable.

_ _ _ _

_ _ _ _

_ _ _ _

_ _ _ _

_ _ _ _

_ _ _ _

_ _ _ _

A portion of a natural object.

Arrange in a container.

An unknown and unpredictable phenomenon that leads to a favorable outcome.

A delicate decorative fabric woven in an open web of symmetrical patterns.

FACE

FROM DEAR TO FOUR

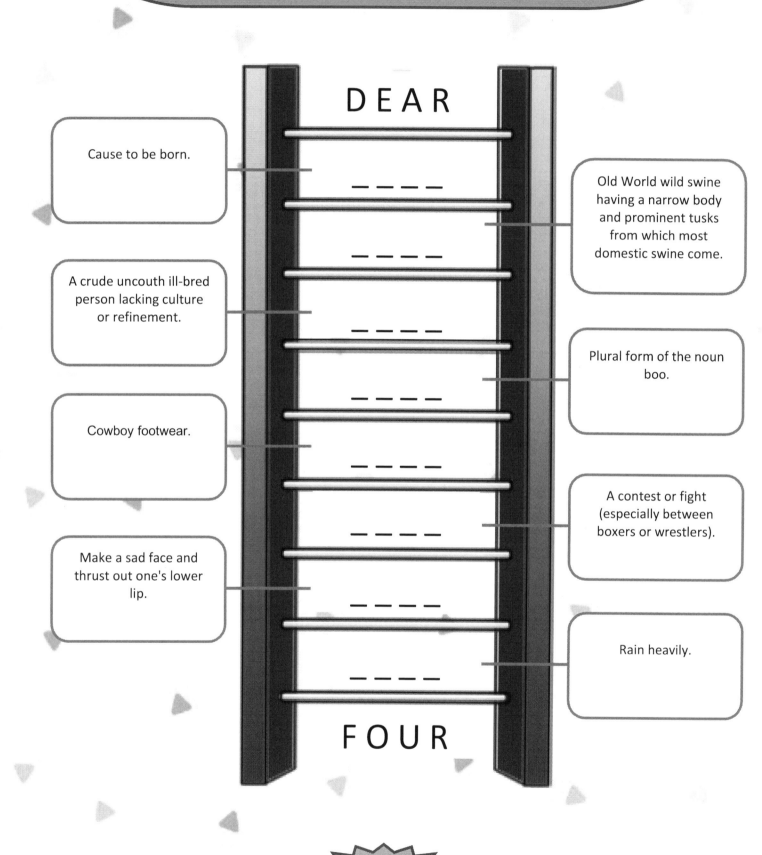

DEAR

Cause to be born.

Old World wild swine having a narrow body and prominent tusks from which most domestic swine come.

A crude uncouth ill-bred person lacking culture or refinement.

Plural form of the noun boo.

Cowboy footwear.

A contest or fight (especially between boxers or wrestlers).

Make a sad face and thrust out one's lower lip.

Rain heavily.

FOUR

FROM WARY TO STUD

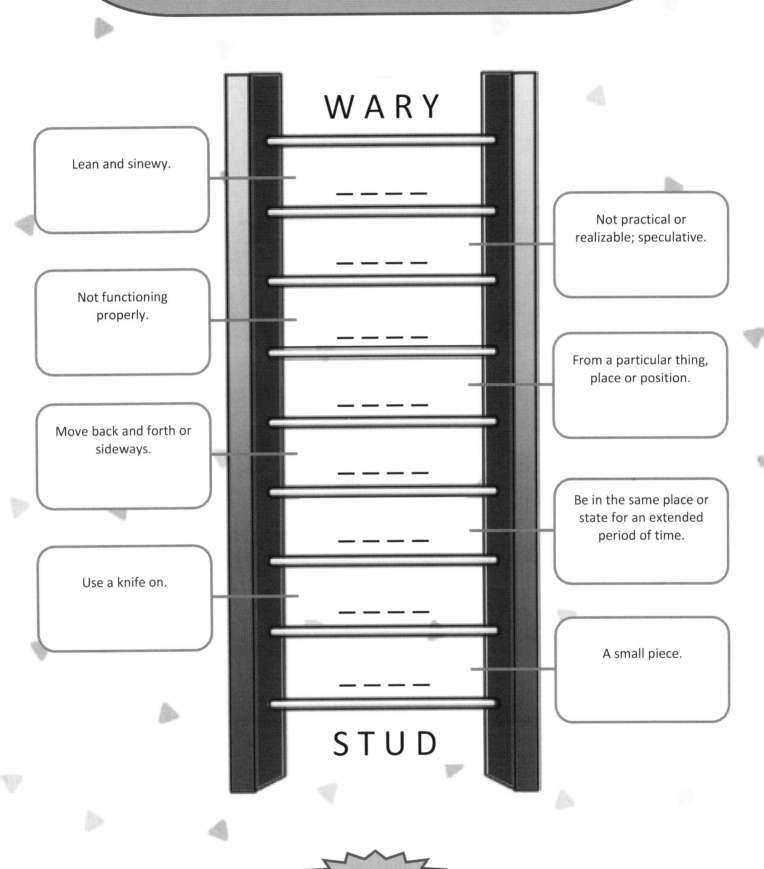

WARY

Lean and sinewy.

Not practical or realizable; speculative.

Not functioning properly.

From a particular thing, place or position.

Move back and forth or sideways.

Be in the same place or state for an extended period of time.

Use a knife on.

A small piece.

STUD

67

FROM FRET TO GRID

FRET

_ _ _ _

_ _ _ _

_ _ _ _

_ _ _ _

_ _ _ _

_ _ _ _

_ _ _ _

GRID

Costing nothing.

Great merriment.

Moody and melancholic.

A metric unit of weight equal to one thousandth of a kilogram.

Run away quickly.

Cement consisting of a sticky substance that is used as an adhesive.

(Informal) glamorous.

A person who has received a degree from a school (high school, college or university).

TAKE

A long thin piece of cloth or paper as used for binding or fastening.

_ _ _ _

Plural form of the noun tap.

_ _ _ _

Plural form of the noun tip.

_ _ _ _

Third-person singular form of the simple present indicative tense of the verb to top.

_ _ _ _

Exclamation used to acknowledge a mistake or accident.

_ _ _ _

Third-person singular form of the simple present indicative tense of the verb to pop.

Plural form of the noun mop.

_ _ _ _

_ _ _ _

Plural form of the noun map.

_ _ _ _

MASS

SAIL

The part of the earth's surface consisting of humus and disintegrated rock.

_ _ _ _

A secular form of gospel that was a major Black musical genre in the 1960s and 1970s.

_ _ _ _

An open-air market in an Arabian city.

_ _ _ _

Hosiery consisting of a cloth covering for the foot.

_ _ _ _

A pustule in an eruptive disease.

_ _ _ _

_ _ _ _

Keep engaged.

Touching with the tongue.

_ _ _ _

_ _ _ _

Feeling nausea; feeling about to vomit.

PICK

FROM DONE TO TAME

DONE

_ _ _ _

_ _ _ _

_ _ _ _

_ _ _ _

_ _ _ _

_ _ _ _

_ _ _ _

TAME

Have supper; eat dinner.

Explosive device that explodes on contact.

A unit of length equal to 1,760 yards or 5,280 feet.

A plant consisting of one or more buildings with facilities for manufacturing.

Mercantile establishment consisting of a carefully landscaped complex of shops representing leading merchandisers.

The lapse of mankind into sinfulness because of the sin of Adam and Eve.

Great in vertical dimension; high in stature.

A fictional story.

FROM RAFT TO FANS

RAFT

A loud bombastic declamation expressed with strong emotion.

_ _ _ _

Hunt or look for; require for a particular reason.

Become smaller.

_ _ _ _

_ _ _ _

Alcoholic drink made by fermenting juice, usually grape juice.

A movable organ for flying (one of a pair).

_ _ _ _

_ _ _ _

(Music) produce tones with the voice.

Simple past tense form of the verb to sing.

_ _ _ _

_ _ _ _

Hollow or grooved tooth of a venomous snake.

FANS

GALA

An outburst (of laughter).

_ _ _ _

Presented in writing or drama or cinema or as a radio or television program.

_ _ _ _

Characteristic of a man.

_ _ _ _

A small congenital pigmented spot on the skin.

_ _ _ _

Change location.

_ _ _ _

Comparative of much; to a greater degree or extent.

_ _ _ _

Deep soft mud in water or slush.

_ _ _ _

A dark region of considerable extent on the surface of the moon.

_ _ _ _

CARE

DENY

Make a depression into. — D E N T

Skillful in physical movements. — D E F T

Lift or elevate. — H E F T

The handle of a weapon or tool. — H A F T

Cause to stop. — H A L T

Draw slowly or heavily. — H A L E

A particular instance of selling. — S A L E

Free from danger or the risk of harm. — S A F E

SATE

FROM BANG TO PACT

BANG

_ _ _ _

_ _ _ _

_ _ _ _

_ _ _ _

_ _ _ _

_ _ _ _

_ _ _ _

_ _ _ _

PACT

A financial institution that accepts deposits and channels the money into lending activities.

Relative status.

A stack of hay.

Select carefully from a group.

Unpleasantly cool and humid.

Building that contains a surface for ice skating or roller skating.

Strike with the foot.

Fill to capacity.

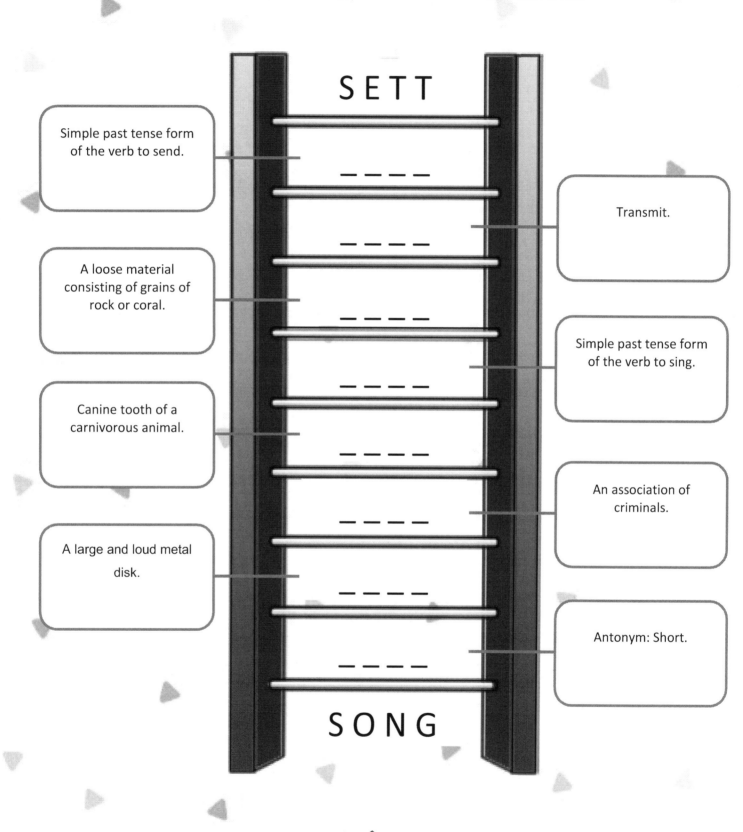

SETT

Simple past tense form of the verb to send.

Transmit.

A loose material consisting of grains of rock or coral.

Simple past tense form of the verb to sing.

Canine tooth of a carnivorous animal.

An association of criminals.

A large and loud metal disk.

Antonym: Short.

SONG

FROM LAST TO GNAW

LAST

The time that has elapsed.

After; later.

_ _ _ _

_ _ _ _

Make a sad face and thrust out one's lower lip.

Cause to flee.

_ _ _ _

_ _ _ _

A contest or fight (especially between boxers or wrestlers).

Gout is a disease which causes people's joints to swell painfully, especially in their toes.

_ _ _ _

The tenth sign of the zodiac; the sun is in this sign from about December 22 to January 19.

Any of various small biting flies: midges; biting midges; black flies; sand flies

_ _ _ _

GNAW

BUCK

Play music in a public place and solicit money for it.

_ _ _ _

A large wilderness area.

_ _ _ _

An uproarious party.

_ _ _ _

Clean one's body by immersion into water.

_ _ _ _

A solemn promise, usually invoking a divine witness, regarding your future acts or behavior.

_ _ _ _

Number science.

_ _ _ _

A fellow member of a team.

_ _ _ _

A line that indicates a boundary.

_ _ _ _

MERE

FROM TEXT TO FEEL

TEXT

The small projection of a mammary gland.

_ _ _ _

The flesh of animals (including fishes and birds and snails) used as food.

Made of fermented honey and water.

_ _ _ _

Antonym: Alive.

Two items of the same kind.

_ _ _ _

(used of color) artificially produced; not natural.

Something that people do or cause to happen.

_ _ _ _

Give food to.

_ _ _ _

FEEL

FROM RUNG TO HULK

RUNG

_ _ _ _

Simple past tense form of the verb to ring.

When somebody is calling you. Your phone will ____.

_ _ _ _

A sheet of ice prepared for playing certain sports, such as hockey or curling.

_ _ _ _

Slender-bodied semiaquatic mammal having partially webbed feet; valued for its fur.

_ _ _ _

A white nutritious liquid secreted by mammals and used as food by human beings.

_ _ _ _

A fabric made from the fine threads produced by certain insect larvae.

_ _ _ _

A mood or display of sullen aloofness or withdrawal.

_ _ _ _

The property possessed by a large mass.

_ _ _ _

HULK

FROM SITS TO SEAL

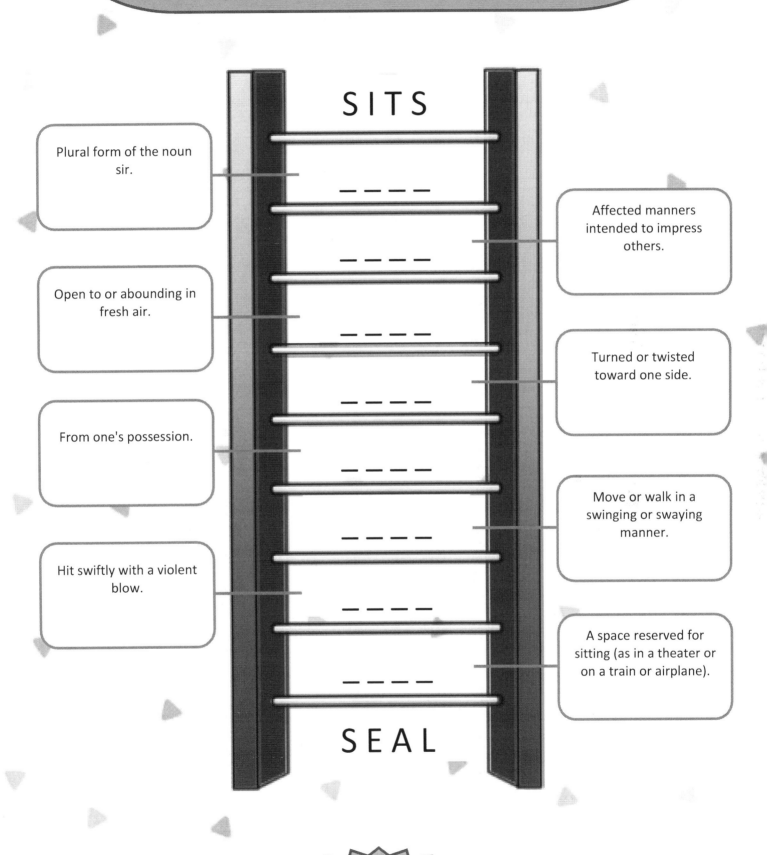

SITS

Plural form of the noun sir.

Affected manners intended to impress others.

Open to or abounding in fresh air.

Turned or twisted toward one side.

From one's possession.

Move or walk in a swinging or swaying manner.

Hit swiftly with a violent blow.

A space reserved for sitting (as in a theater or on a train or airplane).

SEAL

FROM FLEE TO GLOM

FLEE

Simple past tense form of the verb to flee. — _ _ _ _

Winter ride. — _ _ _ _

Get rid of. — _ _ _ _

Wearing footgear. — _ _ _ _

Give evidence of, as of records. — _ _ _ _

Precipitation falling from clouds in the form of ice crystals. — _ _ _ _

Not moving quickly. — _ _ _ _

Shine intensely, as if with heat. — _ _ _ _

GLOM

AWED

Simple past tense form of the verb to owe.

Third-person singular form of the simple present indicative tense of the verb to owe.

Third-person singular form of the simple present indicative tense of the verb to own.

Plural form of the noun owl.

Plural form of the noun oil.

Plural form of the noun mil.

Seminal fluid produced by male fish.

A lager of high alcohol content; by law it is considered too alcoholic to be sold as lager or beer.

SALT

FROM RIND TO GASH

RIND

_ _ _ _

_ _ _ _

_ _ _ _

_ _ _ _

_ _ _ _

_ _ _ _

_ _ _ _

GASH

A team in the sports of curling or bowls.

Any of two families of small parasitic arachnids with barbed proboscis; feed on blood of warm-blooded animals.

Spread manure, as for fertilization.

The ratio of the speed of a moving body to the speed of sound.

[Brit] A painful muscle spasm especially in the neck or back.

Fit snugly into.

A great deal; very.

Reduce to small pieces or particles by pounding or abrading.

FROM OOPS TO BEET

OOPS

_ _ _ _

Plural form of the noun top.

Lots of something.

_ _ _ _

Plural form of the noun toe.

_ _ _ _

Plural form of the noun tee.

_ _ _ _

Simple past tense form of the verb to tee.

_ _ _ _

Increase or justify; supply with a source of material.

_ _ _ _

Plural form of the noun fee.

_ _ _ _

Plural form of the noun bee.

_ _ _ _

BEET

FROM HUNG TO MOLE

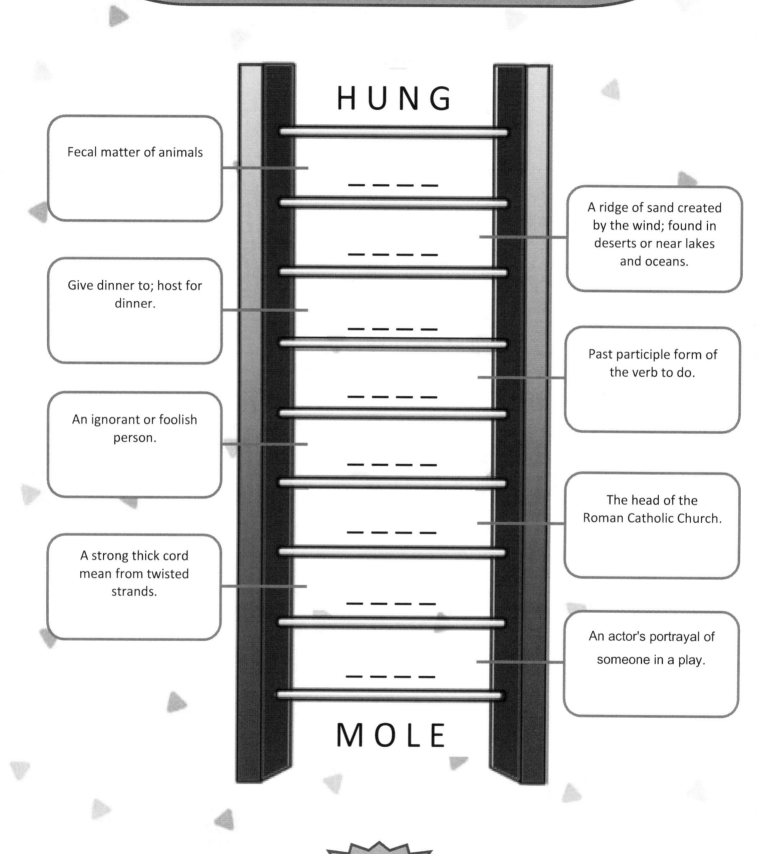

HUNG

Fecal matter of animals

A ridge of sand created by the wind; found in deserts or near lakes and oceans.

Give dinner to; host for dinner.

Past participle form of the verb to do.

An ignorant or foolish person.

The head of the Roman Catholic Church.

A strong thick cord mean from twisted strands.

An actor's portrayal of someone in a play.

MOLE

BLEU

Simple past tense form of the verb to blow.

Simple past tense form of the verb to fly.

_ _ _ _

(Often followed by 'of') a large number, amount or extent.

_ _ _ _

(Cooking) cook slowly and for a long time in liquid.

_ _ _ _

Fill by packing tightly.

_ _ _ _

_ _ _ _

Antonym: Go.

The act of changing location by raising the foot and setting it down.

_ _ _ _

Printing: cancel, as of a correction or deletion.

_ _ _ _

STEW

FROM TINT TO PORE

TINT

_ _ _ _

_ _ _ _

_ _ _ _

_ _ _ _

_ _ _ _

_ _ _ _

_ _ _ _

PORE

Any north temperate plant of the genus Mentha with aromatic leaves and small mauve flowers.

Seek, search for.

Throw forcefully.

Be or become preserved.

Make an indirect suggestion.

Give trouble or pain to.

Form a curl or kink.

Free of extraneous elements of any kind.

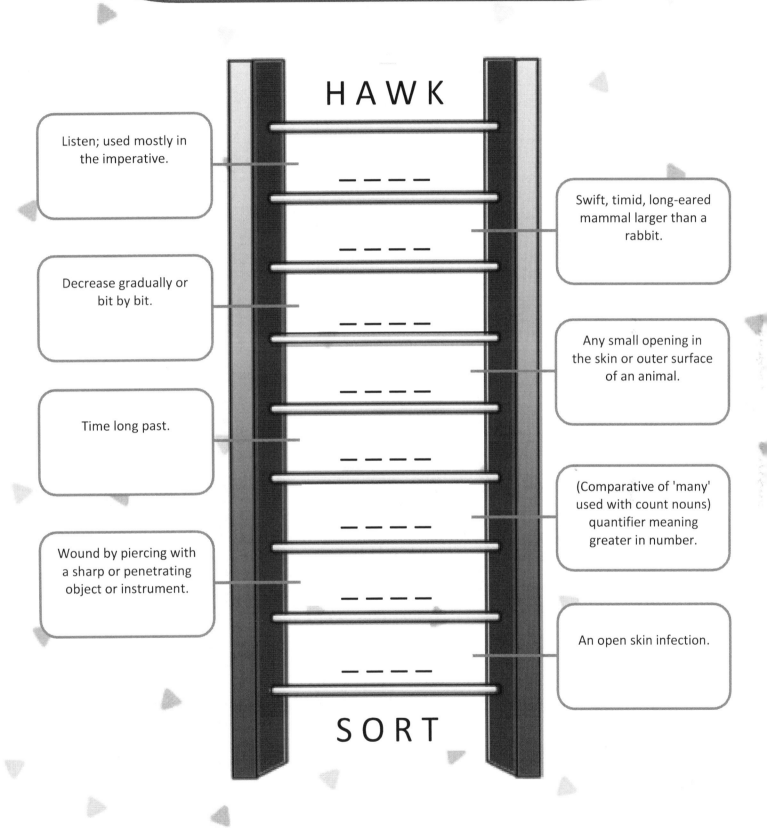

HAWK

Listen; used mostly in the imperative.

Swift, timid, long-eared mammal larger than a rabbit.

Decrease gradually or bit by bit.

Any small opening in the skin or outer surface of an animal.

Time long past.

(Comparative of 'many' used with count nouns) quantifier meaning greater in number.

Wound by piercing with a sharp or penetrating object or instrument.

An open skin infection.

SORT

PART

A sheltered area of coast where ships can dock or anchor safely.

_ _ _ _

(Law) any wrongdoing for which an action for damages may be brought.

(Of food) pleasantly sharp or acid.

_ _ _ _

A male deer, especially an adult male red deer.

Cause emotional anguish or make miserable.

_ _ _ _

Make a thrusting forward movement.

The frame or body of ship.

_ _ _ _

A very large person; impressive in size or qualities.

_ _ _ _

BULK

ANSWERS

1. FIST, FAST, VAST, VASE, VALE, VILE, FILE, FILL

2. CRASS, BRASS, BRATS, BEATS, BEANS, BEADS, BENDS, BONDS

3. LUMP, LIMP, LIME, LINE, LONE, BONE, BOND, BOLD

4. BUNCH, BENCH, BEACH, PEACH, PEACE, PLACE, PLANE, PLANS

5. SLIM, SLID, SAID, SAIL, SOIL, BOIL, BOLL, BOLD

6. CITY, CITE, MITE, MILE, MILD, MOLD, GOLD, GOOD

7. FREE, FRET, FEET, FELT, FELL, FALL, MALL, TALL

8. SLED, SLEW, SLOW, GLOW, GROW, BROW, BREW, DREW

9. GREED, GRASS, TREED, TREES, TRESS, CRESS, CRASS, BRASS

10. WARM, WORM, WORD, WOLD, COLD, FOLD, MOLD, MOLE

11. SELL, SEAL, SEAR, STAR, SPAR, SPUR, SLUR, BLUR

12. TRIPS, GRIPS, GRITS, WRITS, WAITS, WARTS, FARTS, FAITH

13. WIDE, WINE, WIND, FIND, MIND, MILD, MILL, WILL

14. DID, DIE, TIE, TIP, PIP, POP, POT, PET

15. FLAT, FLAG, SLAG, SLUG, SLUR, SOUR, FOUR, FOUL

16. BITS, BIOS, BOOS, MOOS, MOON, BOON, BORN, BORE

17. LIFT, LIFE, WIFE, WISE, RISE, ROSE, ROLE, SOLE

18. TRAM, TEAM, TEAK, PEAK, PECK, PUCK, LUCK, BUCK

19. BOOK, COOK, ROOK, ROOD, FOOD, FOND, FEND, LEND

20. GLUE, GLUT, GOUT, POUT, PORT, PART, PANT, PINT

21. TEAL, REAL, READ, BEAD, BEAT, BOAT, BOOT, BOOK

22. PATH, PATS, PITS, PIUS, PLUS, PLUM, SLUM, SLAM

23. WIND, MIND, MINT, MIST, MISS, KISS, KITS, KITE

24. SMITE, SKITE, SKATE, SLATE, BLATE, BLATS, BEATS, BEARS

25. SKID, SAID, SAND, BAND, LAND, LEND, BEND, SEND

26. GULL, GULP, PULP, PUMP, HUMP, HEMP, HEAP, REAP

27. PLATE, PLANE, PLACE, GLACE, GRACE, TRACE, TRUCE, TRUCK

28. RAID, SAID, SAND, WAND, WIND, FIND, FINE, MINE

29. CHINS, CHINK, CLINK, SLINK, SLICK, SNICK, SNECK, SNEAK

30. SLIP, SLAP, SLOP, SLOT, BLOT, BOOT, BOUT, POUT

31. HOED, HEED, HEAD, HEAP, REAP, REAR, BEAR, TEAR

32. BATE, LATE, LATH, LASH, LASE, LOSE, POSE, POSY

33. SLOT, BLOT, BLOC, BLOW, GLOW, GROW, GREW, DREW

34. ABED, ACED, ACID, ARID, GRID, GRIN, GAIN, MAIN

35. GONG, GONE, TONE, TONS, TOWS, TOWN, DOWN, DAWN

36. BOAST, ROAST, ROUST, ROUSE, BOUSE, BOULE, BOGLE, BOGIE

37. DRAW, DREW, GREW, GROW, GLOW, BLOW, BLOG, SLOG

38. NARY, MARY, MIRY, AIRY, AIRS, AIMS, ARMS, ARMY

39. SHEAF, SHEAR, SPEAR, SPEAK, SPECK, SPICK, SLACK, STICK

40. BRAVE, GRAVE, GRADE, GLADE, GLIDE, GUIDE, GUILE, GUILT

41. PINK, PINS, PIUS, PLUS, FLUS, FLUE, BLUE, CLUE

42. CREST, BREST, BLEST, BLENT, BLUNT, BLUET, BLUES, FLUES

43. SETTLE, SETTEE, SETTER, BETTER, BATTER, FATTER, FALTER, FILTER

44. WINDER, WANDER, WARDER, HARDER, HARPER, HAMPER, HAMMER, HUMMER

45. ROUTE, ROUTS, ROOTS, BOOTS, BLOTS, BLOCS, BLOCK, CLOCK

46. POSE, PORE, CORE, CURE, CUTE, MUTE, MUTT, PUTT

47. GINS, BINS, BITS, BITE, BATE, FATE, DATE, LATE

48. SAME, SANE, WANE, WANT, PANT, PANE, PALE, MALE

ANSWERS

49. MANE, MANO, MONO, MONK, MOCK, SOCK, SUCK, SUCH

50. ROOTS, COOTS, COONS, COINS, CHINS, CHINK, CHICK, CHECK

51. SURF, SERF, SELF, SELL, SILL, SILD, SIND, SEND

52. MATE, MATS, OATS, ORTS, ORBS, ORES, OWES, OWED

53. SPAR, SPAN, SPIN, SPIT, SUIT, QUIT, QUID, QUIN

54. LEAD, LOAD, LOAM, ROAM, ROAR, BOAR, BOAT, BOLT

55. POMP, ROMP, RAMP, RAMS, RATS, RATE, BATE, BALE

56. HURT, CURT, CART, CARE, CAFE, CAME, SAME, TAME

57. PLAT, SLAT, SPAT, SPOT, SHOT, SHOP, SHIP, SHIN

58. CURD, CORD, WORD, WOOD, WOOL, POOL, FOOL, FOUL

59. KINK, PINK, PINT, PANT, PANE, PALE, WALE, WALL

60. BEAR, BEER, BEET, FEET, FEED, SEED, SPED, SLED

61. MURK, MUSK, MASK, MAST, MATT, MUTT, MUTE, CUTE

62. REAM, BEAM, TEAM, TEEM, TEED, TOED, HOED, HOOD

63. LEAF, LEAT, LEAK, PEAK, PEEK, REEK, LEEK, LEET

64. RUNE, RUSE, RUSH, LURK, RASP, GASP, GAMP, GAME

65. PORT, PART, PACT, PACK, PUCK, LUCK, LACK, LACE

66. BEAR, BOAR, BOOR, BOOS, BOOT, BOUT, POUT, POUR

67. WIRY, AIRY, AWRY, AWAY, SWAY, STAY, STAB, STUB

68. FREE, FLEE, GLEE, GLUE, GLUM, GLAM, GRAM, GRAD

69. TAPE, TAPS, TIPS, TOPS, OOPS, POPS, MOPS, MAPS

70. SOIL, SOUL, SOUK, SOCK, POCK, LOCK, LICK, SICK

71. DINE, MINE, MILE, MILL, MALL, FALL, TALL, TALE

72. RANT, WANT, WANE, WINE, WING, SING, SANG, FANG

ANSWERS

73. GALE, TALE, MALE, MOLE, MOVE, MORE, MIRE, MARE

74. DENT, DEFT, HEFT, HAFT, HALT, HALE, SALE, SAFE

75. BANK, DANK, RANK, RINK, RICK, KICK, PICK, PACK

76. SENT, SEND, SAND, SANG, FANG, GANG, GONG, LONG

77. PAST, POST, POUT, ROUT, BOUT, GOUT, GOAT, GNAT

78. BUSK, BUSH, BASH, BATH, OATH, MATH, MATE, METE

79. TEAT, MEAT, MEAD, DEAD, DYAD, DYED, DEED, FEED

80. RANG, RING, RINK, MINK, MILK, SILK, SULK, BULK

81. SIRS, AIRS, AIRY, AWRY, AWAY, SWAY, SWAT, SEAT

82. FLED, SLED, SHED, SHOD, SHOW, SNOW, SLOW, GLOW

83. OWED, OWES, OWNS, OWLS, OILS, MILS, MILT, MALT

84. RINK, RICK, TICK, TUCK, MUCK, MUCH, MACH, MASH

85. TOPS, TONS, TOES, TEES, TEED, FEED, FEES, BEES

86. DUNG, DUNE, DINE, DONE, DOPE, POPE, ROPE, ROLE

87. BLEW, FLEW, SLEW, STEW, STOW, STOP, STEP, STET

88. MINT, HINT, HUNT, HURT, HURL, CURL, CURE, PURE

89. HARK, HARE, PARE, PORE, YORE, MORE, GORE, SORE

90. PORT, TORT, TART, HART, HURT, HURL, HULL, HULK

Conclusion

Thank you again for buying this book! I hope you enjoyed with my book. Finally, if you like this book, please take the time to share your thoughts and post a review on Amazon. It'd be greatly appreciated! Thank you!

Next Steps
– Write me an honest review about the book –
I truly value your opinion and thoughts and I will incorporate
them into my next book, which is already underway.

Get more free bonus here

www.funspace.club
Follow us : facebook.com/funspaceclub

Made in the USA
Columbia, SC
05 June 2022